Managing Menopause Beautifully

MANAGING MENOPAUSE BEAUTIFULLY

Physically, Emotionally, and Sexually

Dona Caine-Francis, NP, CNS

Sex, Love, and Psychology
Judy Kuriansky, Series Editor

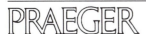

Westport, Connecticut
London

Library of Congress Cataloging-in-Publication Data

Caine-Francis, Dona.
   Managing menopause beautifully : physically, emotionally, and
sexually / Dona Caine-Francis.
       p. cm. — (Sex, love, and psychology, ISSN 1554–222X)
   Includes bibliographical references and index.
   ISBN 978–0–313–34824–2 (alk. paper)
  1. Menopause—Popular works. I. Title.
   RG186.C25   2008
   618.1'75—dc22   2008018049

British Library Cataloguing in Publication Data is available.

Library of Congress Catalog Card Number: 2008018049
ISBN: 978–0–313–34824–2
ISSN: 1554–222X

First published in 2008

Praeger Publishers, 88 Post Road West, Westport, CT 06881
An imprint of Greenwood Publishing Group, Inc.
www.praeger.com

Printed in the United States of America

The paper used in this book complies with the
Permanent Paper Standard issued by the National
Information Standards Organization (Z39.48–1984).

10 9 8 7 6 5 4 3 2 1

*To today's seasoned women who have committed to sharing the
"magic of menopause" with their daughters and granddaughters
the seasoned women of tomorrow!*

CONTENTS

FOREWORD

Whenever I hear complaints about women getting older or going through "the change of life," I remember what Gloria Steinem said to someone expressing surprise at how fit Gloria looked then at 50. "This is what 50 looks like," she said proudly. Now every woman can respond as Gloria did, at 50, 60, or any age, armed with the guidance in Dona Caine-Francis's present book, *Managing Menopause Beautifully*. As Dona encourages us, feel your most confident and keep yourself healthy—physically, emotionally, sexually, and spiritually—and you can not only proudly announce your age but also live your life to the fullest as a "seasoned woman."

Of course, there are changes that come with "the change." But in these pages, Dona alerts us about what to expect and how to prepare ourselves so that menopause is not a "pause" at all but rather a reenergizing. Reinvent yourself, Dona implores us—reminding me of the secret to rock star Madonna's fountain of vitality by being the "Queen of Reinvention" even as she turned 50 years old. Make yourself anew, and you will never feel old.

For every woman going through the change of life at any age, Dona's book should be by her side as well as that of all her friends, family, and health professionals who care for her.

Dona's book is full of need-to-know facts as well as alternative strategies, personal stories, myth busting, and helpful relationship and intimacy scales. After so many years of answering women's questions—on radio and television and through my newspaper and magazine columns—I knew when I met Dona at the American Association of Sexuality Educators, Counselors and

Therapists that she was one to join in answering these questions and providing support and guidance to so many women. Her personal glow and enthusiasm to be of service to others is heartwarming. Just as she fulfilled her dream in writing this book, Dona's book will inspire other women to do the same in their own way.

Dr. Judy Kuriansky
Series Editor

ACKNOWLEDGMENTS

This book would not have been possible without the courageous clients who have shared their stories, challenges, and successes—all of which have sensitized my work and my appreciation for the human spirit. Generally the stories shared have used the term "partner" and for some that may be a same sex partner. My hope is not to offend readers, but open a dialogue for women and partners to share a future of passion and living life well together. These narratives are with the permission of those brave soles who want others to learn from their journey. They are members of the Magnificent Menopause newsletter family. www.magnificentmenopause.com is my Web site offering biweekly articles regarding menopause. Clients ask their questions and often find the answers in the next newsletter. Visit the site and "Ask Dona" your questions!

A special thank you to Judy Kuriansky who introduced me to Debbie Carvalko from Praeger at that monumental AASECT conference in St. Louis. Who would have thought this project would be one of the outcomes of that meeting?

Mary Cotofan and the staff at Apex CoVantage, you are awesome. Thanks to Bruce Owens for managing to clean up a manuscript full of ideas but low on punctuation. You helped make this journey less stressful.

And yet, we do not live these endeavors without the support and sacrifice of family. Brad—my husband, illustrator, friend, and golf partner—I thank you for your patience and support. And yes, I do have a tee time for Saturday. Ben, how could one 22-year-old son manage to know so much about computers? My daughter Jordan, you found those moments to cheer me on and help me see the project with an end in sight. And to Ansley, my physical therapist who helped this perimenopausal woman maintain some motion in that frozen shoulder while spending 10 and 12 hour days at the computer, I say many thanks.

As an author one does not know when the words you share lift another to take that next step. Thank you Gail Sheehy for your belief in the "seasoned woman" and sharing that wonderful view of women to an eager public. May this book take Gail's persona one step further. Ladies, thrive as a seasoned woman and continue challenging society's rules and bending them for our next generation.

Chapter One

MENOPAUSE: PHYSICAL, EMOTIONAL, AND SEXUAL REINVENTION

Life is either a daily adventure or nothing. To keep our faces toward change and behave like a free spirit in the presence of fate is strength undefeatable!

—Helen Keller

The transition into menopause is indeed "a daily adventure." All too often, women face this natural life cycle with confusion, lack of knowledge, conflicting advice, and surprise. Menopause marks the end of a woman's reproductive life. The menopause transition opens a pathway for women to experience hormonal adjustments; the body's response to hormonal fluctuations; a cascade of symptoms, including hot flashes and sleep disruption, two of the more perplexing symptoms; and the emotional shift for a woman as she incorporates this new identity. Our society historically has diminished value for the aging woman, whereas in other cultures the aging woman is a sage, leader, healer, and mentor. Western culture assigns menopause as the downhill course of aging—sagging skin, wrinkles, the cessation of sexuality, and a decrease in mental functioning—the beginning of "the end."

"No way, not me," I say. I proclaim a different path for myself not only as a woman but also as a psychotherapist, nurse practitioner, and sex therapist. With my clients, I have witnessed something different than this age-old prophecy. Their questions, struggles, challenges, successes, and strength bring forth other options for today's seasoned woman.

Menopause is a metamorphosis, and it is different for each woman regardless of how her mother or sister handled the "change." Like puberty, menopause is not necessarily fun, but the end result is maturity and growth. I would like to challenge women to consider this natural life cycle an opportunity to "reinvent the self" and let that reinvention flow into the physical, emotional, and sexual domains of life. Remember two important points. First, not all women have the cascade of symptoms with their menopause transition, and approximately 20 percent have very few. Studies suggest that the majority, some 50 percent of women, experience a moderate group of symptoms and tolerate them well. It seems that the remaining 30 percent struggle through the passage and generally need some intervention.[1] Second, for many readers, you are at life's halfway mark and can live another 42 years. Your journey is composed of learning experiences, friends and family who have touched you, and accomplishments and disappointments that gather into your book of life and make you who you are. What will the next chapters showcase? Will your legacy be, "She lived life fully"?

Many books on the bookstore shelf talk of the wisdom of menopause and how to achieve the perfect balance and an ageless transition, yet few focus on the emotional and sexual options women have for embracing this phase of life with resilience. My hope is that this book will do just that: provide strategies to enhance your physical stature, emotional vitality, and sexual well-being and some guidelines for your partner so that he or she can be knowledgeable, supportive, and engaged in the process of reinvention with you.

Colleagues have gone before me, sharing their personal stories. I remember in my thirties sitting in an audience at an annual meeting of the American Association of Sexuality Educators, Counselors and Therapists in awe of the speaker, Lonnie Barbach. Her books filled my office shelves. They were in my lending library for clients. And now here I sat, soaking up her words and her spirit and hearing of her recent book *The Pause*.[2] "I wrote this book because I found myself in the menopause life cycle. My insights and investigation are an offering for those women that followed," remarked Lonnie. Never did I imagine that those words would be a calling for me some 20 years later. At the time, I thought how nice of Lonnie to share her story and wisdom, but she doesn't look "that old." Women are wonderful storytellers. I know that to be truth after my years in the nursing profession—the stories told of patients, their families, and the monumental courage and wisdom they have taught each nurse as we advocate and care for them.

Managing Menopause is more the stories from clients in my private practice than my personal story. I may slip a few anecdotes in here and there. More than 30 years in nursing opens many doors for stories. The challenge of an open-heart-surgery unit in the 1970s, a busy emergency room in Las Vegas, Boston's influence on a young master's degree student, directing an emergency medicine department in rural Maine, managing a psychiatric unit in North Carolina, and growing several psychotherapy practices in North Carolina—all of these settings usher in multiple scenarios.

GENERATION INFLUENCES

An estimated 60 million American women are somewhere in the menopause transition or postmenopausal. In 2006, the first group of baby-boomer women (1946–1964) turned age 60 with an average of 6,000 women a day entering menopause in the United States.[3] These women are a growing population who are no longer silent or invisible. They are well educated, vocal, and sophisticated and choose to be decision makers for their health care. Don't I know this to be a fact? Men and women enter my office with statistics, articles, and medication reviews in their hands, wanting to know if this could help their symptoms or be their diagnosis. Demanding clear, accurate information and options for symptom relief can only reshape the health care system and demand that health care providers include the consumer in "shared-decision-making" models for care.

Parents of boomers, the Veteran generation, born from 1922 to 1945 (see Table 1.1), have a different posture regarding menopause and options for care. The youngest, now age 63, lived in the era of silence for the menopausal woman, possess an appreciation for authority, and are now grandmothers. Many may encourage their daughters to seek appropriate care even though they managed menopause with the quick fix offered by their physicians (hysterectomy) and remain on the same initial doses of hormones. It is the grandmother role that brings them out of silence. They do not want their grandchildren to be patronized, silenced, or dismissed regarding their hormonal concerns.

Baby boomers—those born between 1946 and 1964—were the first generation to be raised on television. Ideal family systems were portrayed in the television programs *Leave It to Beaver* and *Father Knows Best*. Real-life events influenced the mind-set of baby boomers—the man on the moon, the Vietnam War, protests over the draft, the sexual revolution, the civil rights movement, gay rights, the environmental movement, women's liberation and birth control, rock and roll, hallucinogenic drugs, and recreational drug use.[4] It is no wonder that the boomer generation developed a voice and presence and entered every life cycle leaving them vastly different. They swarmed schools with their numbers. Guidance counselors in high school brought forth other vocations for

Table 1.1
Generation Time Line

Veterans	Born 1922–1945
Baby boomers	Born 1946–1964
Generation X	Born 1965–1978
Generation Y	Born 1979–1995

women beyond the typical nursing, teacher, secretary, and homemaker options. College life, as it had been known, was imploded with coed dorms, protests, and marching for civil rights. And when they got into the workforce, "glass ceilings" were broken through. Maternity wards became flooded with young women insisting on the presence of their partners, birthing rooms, and other options to bring about more natural childbirth experiences. Waiting to have children until later in life became another option for these pacesetters. Then, in later years, boomers have had to acknowledge that their parents live longer because of modern technology. However, this phenomenon has led to another cultural shift, the "sandwich generation." Adults are caring for both elderly parents and young children at the same time, and now the "aging process" is bombarded with this aggressive, demanding population of baby boomers. Boomer women will not settle for a menopause scenario of wrinkles, power surges, memory lapses, and sexual stall-out. If you are one of the vocal, assertive women described here, then this book is for you.

But what about the generation that follows the baby boomers—Generation X?

Generation X heralds from 1965 to 1978, and the oldest of this generation are age 34. They were influenced by pop culture from the 1980s and witnessed the fall of the Berlin Wall, the end of the Cold War, the explosion of technology, and the post-9/11 world. As young adults, their stereotypical reputation is being self-reliant, cynical, mistrusting of traditional values and institutions, and unimpressed with authority and tech savvy.[5] However, as new parents, their persona has transformed into proactive moms and dads because of the events they experienced. Gratitude must go to Generation X for busting forth with entrepreneurial spirit and their influence on techno-friendly growth and ingenuity. Google, Yahoo!, MySpace, Facebook, Amazon, Dell, and YouTube are a few of their contributions.

Children of baby boomers are the next generation identified. Controversy exists regarding which years and terminology to utilize: Generation Y, echo boomers, or Millennials (born in 1979–1995). They are often labeled as rebellious, rude, demanding, and impatient. Employers praise their energy, charisma, and ability to find information and solve problems.[6] They have grown up digital. A survey by Junco and Mastrodicasa regarding college students and their digital possessions find that the vast majority have computers, cell phones, instant messaging, Web sites, blogs, Facebook accounts, and expensive portable music devices such as iPods.[7] However, a significant shift in demographics should begin in 2011, when the oldest baby boomer (born in 1946) hits 65, the age of legal retirement in the United States. Generation X will make up the middle- and upper-management positions and Generation Y the lower half of the workforce. What needs shall move these next generations into the "seasoned woman" world? Influencing factors such as insistence of ongoing research into women's health, role modeling by boomer women who successfully reinvent themselves, extended life expectancy, and the tenacity of Generations X and Y make the next decade an exciting one to watch.

IGNITE YOUR WELL-BEING

Menopause is a natural part of a woman's life cycle—not a curse, not a medical disorder, not "the beginning of the end" but instead a transition. Yet few women heard this description from their mothers, the media, health care providers, or their partners until recently. The baby-boomer generation benefits from the departure of doom and gloom and the acceleration of new knowledge and new options for women entering menopause. Another significant factor for this generation is the increased life expectancy for boomer women. In general, life expectancy rose rapidly in the twentieth century because of improvements in public health, nutrition, and medicine. It is proposed that life expectancy will continue to increase if death rates from diseases such as heart disease, cancer, hypertension, and diabetes continue to decline. And what of the newest and fastest-growing segment of our population, centenarians, or those who have attained the age of 100 years or more? Currently, there are about 40,000 centenarians in the United States, or a little more than 1 per 10,000 in the population; 85 percent are women, and 15 percent are men.[8] Worldwide there are 450,000 centenarians, and by 2050 "the number of US centenarians is expected to reach 834,000 and maybe even 1 million," said Dr. Robert Butler, president of the International Longevity Center in New York City.[9]

Thus, it is reasonable to suggest that many women will live some 30 to 40 years beyond menopause, a time of vibrancy and excitement and an opportunity to reinvent the "self." As a therapist, I have spent decades encouraging people to tap into their authentic selves, to challenge the past and push beyond resentments or disappointments. Many women find themselves now

Table 1.2
Life Expectancy

	Overall Population	Men	Women
United Nations worldwide	67.2 years	65.0	69.5
U.S. data (ranked 38th in United Nations)	78.2 years	75.6	80.8

Source: CIA World Factbook, 2008.

with time and energy that isn't claimed by responsibility for others. Women describe this life phase as invigorating and promising, with new opportunities in family life, interests, friendships, creative outlets, relationships with a partner or spouse, a new definition of self, and maybe a chance to rekindle the youthful spirit of long ago.

All of this is good news for our health, longevity, and well-being. And since most women transition into menopause somewhere between the ages 35 and 58 with the median age of 52, we have a lot of living to do postmenopause. Kenneth Manton, research professor of demographic studies at Duke University, says that a healthy woman who reaches age 50 free of cancer and heart disease can expect to see her ninety-second birthday.[10]

Demographer's report that Americans are taking longer to grow up and much longer to die, shifting all stages of adulthood by at least 10 years. So how do you receive this information regarding your longevity—with excitement, puzzlement, and dread or with whimsy and determination?

Gail Sheehy, in her book *Sex and the Seasoned Woman: Pursing the Passionate Life*, writes of the passage from first adulthood to second adulthood and the potential that awaits the seasoned woman. Her message validates much of what I have witnessed recently in my private practice: women who are ready to move beyond life scripts that no longer fit the "woman" they have become. "Often this advancement comes after they have launched their last child, find their selves negotiating a serious illness, dealing with the upheaval of menopause, loss of a close friend through death, or the monumental loss of a lifelong mate via death or divorce."[11] My hope is that readers in early stages of perimenopause will seize the moment and begin to script their passage in a proactive manner.

This increased life span presents a blank slate. What you write on the blank slate in second adulthood is what makes the difference. Sheehy portrays first adulthood as surviving by figuring out how to "please and perform" for the powerful people who protect and reward: parents, teachers, mates, and bosses. By the mid-forties, the trend in second adulthood is to look for greater mastery over the environment—emotional, physical, or vocational—and less fear to speak your voice.[12] How will you reawaken life? A new dream, a spiritual focus, a new passion, a new vocation, a romantic energy for that twenty 20-year-old relationship—where does the turning point lead you?

Passage into second adulthood from my perspective ignites your well-being and quality of life. Many consider "happiness" integral to well-being. Many clients enter the therapy world looking for increased happiness. They associate terms such as "well-being" and "satisfaction" with happiness. In the broadest sense, well-being is a measure of emotional, social, and economic factors as well as happiness, art, and environmental health, which make well-being more difficult to measure.

A subjective index of well-being is but one facet of the issue. People can identify their state of well-being; however, without acknowledging options and establishing a plan, well-being can remain elusive. I often say to clients, "Your awareness is but the first step to change. It is a four-step proposition. First, the awareness; second, identification of options; third, establishing a plan of action; and, last, evaluating the effectiveness of your plan."

I challenge you, too. Ignite your well-being at this junction in life by assessing your well-being. Are you spending too much time in one particular area of life with little positive outcome? Are you at a turning point in life because of situations outside your control, such as the loss of a job, the onset of a disease, or a child moving out to attend college? What are you doing to open new life opportunities for yourself? Are symptoms of perimenopause decreasing your quality of life? It may be time to visit your health care provider with a list of health concerns, including what you have tried, what you have read about, and, now, what you want to put into action. Chapter 4 lists some suggestions to assist you in your partnership with your health care provider. You want someone who is open to your input—one who can give you the time and listen to your concerns. You may already have a provider on your team, but if you don't, I have included a few tips. Well-being is not that elusive. And truly, you are in the driver's seat to enhance your quality of life. Be reflective; take some time to focus on your physical, emotional, and sexual self. Where do you want to be in three to five years? What do you need to do to get there? This book offers today's woman a closer look at three critical domains in life and provides realistic strategies to promote your well-being. The rest, execution, is up to you.

Chapter Two

MENOPAUSE BASICS: WHAT IS HAPPENING TO MY BODY?

The way I see it, if you want the rainbow, you gotta put up with the rain.

—Dolly Parton

Today's woman has at her fingertips far more information about menopause than their mothers had. To make my point, go to your computer (a tool your mother did not have) and search for the term "menopause." How many pages appear under this heading? You will have more than 100 Web sites at your fingertips—a cadre of scientific, treatment, and research sites all offering you information and options for herbal relief and hormone therapy. Next, go to the Amazon site and type in "menopause books." More than 762 books are chronicled for your exploration into the world of menopause. If your mother had been interested enough to do research, she would have had to drive to the library or bookstore, and how many renderings would she have found? Another difference in this generation's access to menopause is the fact you can talk about the subject at lunch with colleagues, at a dinner party with friends, and in other arenas without the fear of upsetting someone or being ignored. The Veteran generation women were told that "it is all in your head" and asked, "When are you going to be your old self again?" or encouraged to just "suck it up." Options for your health and well-being during the menopause transition are plentiful. You need not be silent. It does require your awareness of the normal process of menopause and when it has become more of a distress in your life than a passage. After awareness, the next requirement is your voice—a voice to share the concerns with a health care professional and discuss options to enhance living, not merely to survive. The options include lifestyle changes, herbal supplements, hormone therapy (HT), bioidentical hormones, and strategies to promote your well-being during the transition into menopause and the postmenopause years.

Although the transition into menopause is completely normal because it marks the end of a woman's period of fertility, it can receive mixed reviews. For some, menopause is welcomed and even liberating from the monthly periods and need for contraceptive interventions to prevent pregnancy. Other women may experience menopause with grief, especially if their childbearing years were short or they were not able to conceive. And another population of women have induced menopause from surgery to remove the ovaries, from chemotherapy, and from pelvic radiation. For some women, the unexpected introduction and loss of fertility can be an extremely negative development. Your ability to sort out your feelings regarding the end of fertility, manage the symptoms, choose appropriate treatments, and consciously embrace the upcoming years of potential vitality is up to you. I believe that "attitude" is the enhancing feature for life changes. If you have maintained a fairly positive attitude with previous adjustments in life, such as marriage, child rearing, career adjustment, and health changes, your chances of sustaining that perspective with menopause are good.

The previous generation was caught up in the mystique of menopause and a "no-talk" cultural edict. That provided a forum for ignorance and myths. What are some of the myths that society has perpetuated for women in this aging process? Let me share five of the more common myths regarding menopause.

MYTH 1: SEX STOPS WHEN YOU ENTER MENOPAUSE

Sexual researchers Masters and Johnson found that libido is not solely linked to estrogen levels and thus does not automatically crash during menopause. In fact, most clinicians agree that a woman's sex drive, or libido, has a greater association with testosterone and, further, that the drive to be sexual and the ability to function sexually are also dependent on nonhormonal factors, such as relationships, level of stress, and health. A 1998 survey by the North American Menopause Society of postmenopausal women revealed that 43 percent were happiest and more fulfilled from the ages of 50 to 65 than in earlier years. The majority (51%) noted no difference in their sexual relationships.[1]

Another large study, the Massachusetts Women's Health Study, showed that a woman's menopause status was less significant a deterrent for sexual function than her health, her partner's health, psychological and financial issues, and lifestyle.[2] Yes, hormonal levels can affect sexual desire, arousal, and function, but it is important for women to include relationship and life issues in the equation for sexual well-being.

And for some seasoned sirens, sex can be better than before. Postmenopausal women do not worry about getting pregnant. Often, the kids are out of the house, so more freedom exists to try different times, places, and positions and to add fantasy options. A woman's voice may be stronger, and many know the type of pleasure they enjoy and are not afraid to share their sexual needs. Chapter 8 offers strategies to enhance desire (which may be limping along through menopause), exercises to recapture the lust of seasons past, and "maybe" experiences to help move beyond an automatic "no" for sex.

MYTH 2: MENOPAUSE BEGINS IN YOUR FIFTIES

Perimenopausal symptoms can start in your thirties or anytime menopause is induced by artificial means, such as surgery or chemotherapy. The age is less an issue; rather, the symptoms are propelled by a drop in estrogen and progesterone, two of the sex hormones. Thus, the onset is dependent on one's biochemistry and health status.

Early menopause can also be produced by autoimmune disorders, poor nutrition, and chronic stress where the adrenal glands are constantly being taxed. Most women transition into menopause between the ages of 35 and 58 with the average onset at age 52. Yes, the passage can be a bit of a journey since it can begin 10 to 15 years before your final menstrual period.

MYTH 3: ONCE YOU ARE IN MENOPAUSE, YOU HAVE TO TAKE HORMONES

Another untruth. Hormone therapy depends on the individual and the distress of the symptoms. In fact, a recent study revealed that 20 percent of perimenopausal women experience no physical change other than a gradual cessation of the menstrual cycle; 10 percent are temporarily incapacitated, and 70 percent have moderate symptoms that come and go over a number of years.[3]

Women need to weigh the benefits and risks of taking HT. Women with a history of breast or cervical cancer, high blood pressure, and other medical issues in the family need to carefully assess the risks. However, other options exist to aid those inconvenient symptoms, such as hot flashes, night sweats, and irritability. Remember that, for most, the symptoms of menopause are temporary. Herbal products may be helpful in the short-term treatment. The 30 percent of women with severe symptoms should consult their health care provider and discuss their options for pharmaceutical interventions or even bioidentical hormones made from plants.

MYTH 4: ALL WOMEN SUFFER WITH MENOPAUSE

Some do and some don't. I believe that menopause is as individual as a thumbprint. Talk to your mother or sister about her experience, as she may give you some clues. But so much of your process will depend on you—your nutrition, exercise program, body weight, stress level, and lifestyle. You may be one of the 20 percent who seem to breeze through this life transition. If you are one of the 30 percent with moderate symptoms, perhaps hot flashes during the day minus night sweats or insomnia, some herbal remedies and supplements can help you coast through. My ob-gyn colleagues share stories of perimenopausal women experiencing severe hot flashes and night sweats, researching their options, and asking to try "transdermal patches" with estrogen and progestin to relieve symptoms. These proactive women come into the office well informed with their research in hand prepared to sell their case. A common practice for clinicians is to listen, discuss the risks on the basis of the woman's health and history, identify the benefits of an intervention, start with a low dose for a defined period of time, and then reevaluate hormone levels and her health. Thus, the good news is that menopause and the impacts on your life are manageable. I like to think that you can manage it—beautifully!

MYTH 5: MENOPAUSE GOES ON FOREVER

It may feel like forever, but the reality is that menopause begins when you have gone 12 consecutive months without a period and arrive at the final menstrual period (FMP). The majority of women find that the symptoms experienced in perimenopause are probably improved or resolved in menopause. Yet that 30 percent mentioned previously may still need herbal remedies, bioidenticals, or HT for some time. A part of the bad name that menopause receives is related to the overall aging process. Typically, as individuals age, there are more opportunities for health problems to develop; basic wearing down of the organs and systems of the body result in high blood pressure, heart disease, elevated cholesterol, diabetes, and cancer. Escaping the aging process is a fantasy. Women enter the aging process with a disadvantage if they have smoked, have not exercised regularly, maintained a stable body weight, minimized the impact of stress, and maintained a balanced emotional life. The unpredictable fluctuations in hormones along with natural wear and tear accelerate the aging process for an already vulnerable woman who has not attended to her health.

It is important for women in menopause to reaffirm their commitment to living life well. Now is not the time to neglect your body or take it for granted. As a nurse practitioner, I encourage a few musts for the menopausal woman: monthly self-administered breast exams, annual Pap tests, and screening for colon cancer, cervical cancer, osteoporosis, and heart disease.

MENOPAUSE BASICS

Let's move beyond the fictitious stories assigned to the "change" and focus on menopause basics: what is happening to your body. Menopause comes from the Greek words for "month" and "end," the end of the monthlies. Yet officially menopause is when the monthly periods stop permanently for 12 consecutive months. As menopause approaches, there is an erratic undertone to life. You may be waking up a few times during the night and have difficulty getting back to sleep or possibly not feeling quite like yourself, being more tired and edgy than usual and easy to upset. Your cycle may be a bit longer or shorter and the bleeding somewhat lighter or significantly heavier than usual. But you are only 38—this couldn't be menopause! More women in today's knowledge-based environment recognize that menopause can begin as early as the thirties, and with the environmental estrogens in food products, gynecologists speak of women at age 59 and older who are still menstruating. Just as some young women were bothered by extreme cramping and a monumental flow during puberty as they began their periods, this cessation of the menstrual flow is also individualized. Factors such as stress, diet, exercise, smoking, genetic differences, culture, and self-care skills all affect the menopause transition.

Categories of Menopause States

- Perimenopause

  - Early perimenopause
  - Late perimenopause

- FMP
- Postmenopause

  - Early postmenopause
  - Late postmenopause

- Induced menopause
- Premature menopause

Transitioning into menopause, beginning with the reproductive stage, then through the variable stage of *perimenopause* with its wide and unpredictable fluctuations in hormone production and arriving at the first year of *postmenopause* (early postmenopause) can best be understood by utilizing the STRAW continuum. Figure 2.1 is provided to clarify terms and time frames. This may be helpful in your discussions with health care professionals as you advocate for your health care needs. STRAW offers standardized definitions for the stages of normal reproductive aging in women. The panel of experts who gathered in 2001 to create the nomenclature represented the National Institutes of Health, the North American Menopause Society, and the American Society for Reproductive Medicine. Outlined in Figure 2.1 are the stages, terminology for the stages, duration of a stage, menstrual cycle, and endocrine function. The FMP is the zero (0) point on the graph and falls between late menopause transition (–1), which falls in perimenopause and early postmenopause (+1). Women do not proceed through each stage in a predictable fashion. Some stall in one stage for a considerable period of time, while other women can skip a stage or seesaw back and forth. One recent 54-year-old client of mine has been in early stages of perimenopause for several years. She has longer periods and experiences pronounced flow of her menses, but they remain regular enough that she does not miss a cycle. "I am 54 years old. How much longer can this go on? And the hot flashes do not let up either. My poor husband wears a sweater almost year-round in the house since I keep the house at 68 degrees," she shared at her last session.

A woman "reaches menopause" after 12 consecutive months of absent menstrual cycles that is not caused by illness but by a natural cessation of hormone-produced menstruation. Perimenopause has an early and late state defined by the length of the cycle and an increase in follicle-stimulating hormone (FSH). *Early perimenopause* is technically when the length of your cycle shifts by seven or more days from your norm. *Late perimenopause* is marked by two or more skipped cycles and an absence of menses greater than 60 days. But a woman does not cross the line into menopause until that 12-month absence of flow. Postmenopause, like perimenopause, has an early and late stage. *Early postmenopause,* or stage +1, is defined as the time span within five years after the FMP,

Figure 2.1
Stages of Normal Reproductive Aging in Women

					Final Menstrual Period (FMP)		
Stages:	–5	–4	–3	–2	–1 ▼	+1	+2
Terminology:	Reproductive			Menopausal Transition		Postmenopause	
	Early	Peak	Late	Early	Late*	Early*	Late*
				Perimenopause			
Duration of Stages:	variable			variable		(a) 1 yr / (b) 4 yrs	until demise
Menstrual Cycles:	variable to regular	regular		variable cycle length (> days different from normal)	≥2 skipped cycles and an interval of amenorrhea (≥60 days)	*Amen. x 12 mos* None	
Endocrine:	normal FSH		↑ FSH	↑ FSH		↑ FSH	

*Stages most likely to be characterized by vasomotor symptoms.
Source: Stages of Reproductive Aging Workshop (STRAW), *Menopause,* 2001. North American Menopause Society, *Menopause Practice: A Clinician's Guide,* 3rd ed. (Cleveland, OH: North American Menopause Society, 2007), p. 10.

when ovarian hormone function is dampened even further. One of the scenarios I see in the office describes a woman who was severely bothered by perimenopausal symptoms and was given HT to relieve symptoms. Then, after reaching FMP and entering postmenopause, she required continuation of HT because of insomnia and hot flashes until, on reevaluation of her hormone status and a trial off of medications, she found that she was symptom free. The standard of care when HT is prescribed is to start at a low dose and continue for as short a period of time as necessary, possibly two to three years. Regular evaluation of hormone function with hormone testing is an important element in the HT process. The typical age of a woman reaching menopause is 40 to 58 years. The transition can last 1 to 15 years. Don't panic, though, as typically the transition is about six years. Yet there are cases of women in early postmenopause (within five years of menses cessation) who begin their cycles again. A common finding for this population relates to the intensity of stress, a great loss, or perhaps a significant illness that stresses the body. Take heart—these are not usual cases.

Induced menopause causes a cessation of menstruation from surgical intervention (removal of the ovaries or hysterectomy), chemotherapy, or pelvic radiation. Because a woman is thrust into menopause without the natural fluctuation of hormones, women may have a more pronounced state of symptoms and require support for the disturbance the symptoms bring both physically and emotionally.

Premature menopause occurs in only about 1 percent of women and is marked by spontaneous menopause before a woman is age 40. Possible causes are diabetes, thyroid dysfunction, androgen insufficiency, and rheumatoid arthritis. These women are at greater risk for heart disease, osteoarthritis, and emotional outpouring, especially if the premature nature prevents conception. Now that I have exposed you to more information than many of you needed about the nuances of menopause, I will burden you with an even greater explanation of early hormone function and puberty.

PUBERTY AND HORMONE CHANGES

A surprise is given to you. You knew the time was near for the arrival, but you just thought it would take a little longer. Your womanhood has just taken a huge step. What lies ahead—fun, fear, discomfort, and the glorious opportunities of a new life cycle? Some of you are confused, while others know. I am describing the onset of puberty and that first menstrual cycle. I could also be describing the end of menstrual periods and the possibilities of life beyond the period.

Think back to that time in your life: your first menstrual period. In my day, it was called "your friend." Unless you feared that you might be pregnant, you shouted with glee at the sight of menses. Were you given "the talk" or a "booklet" about the menstrual cycle? Women have been traumatized by a lack of preparation. One client thought that she was bleeding to death until her best friend told her mother, who then called my client's mother to say, "You need to talk to Angela. She thinks she is dying, but it may be her first period!" I want to think that the daughters of baby boomers are better prepared for this phase of womanhood. They have classes at school to prepare them just in case a mother missed that opportunity. Peer groups are not shy; they describe every little detail, and some even brag that they "started" before another. My daughter, Jordan, had no choice but to be educated by her sex therapist mother. I even talked her Girl Scout leaders into having me present a class for the girls at age 10. Although some of the mothers joined their daughters at my house with some reservation, ultimately the girls helped all the moms warm up. I began with an age-appropriate discussion of menstruation and the changes in a girl's body. Then I shared some of the products available to them, from tampons to pads. We had a bowl in the middle of the table to allow any girl to anonymously ask questions. The questions that were asked challenged even my poker face. Pregnancy, oral sex, and "Could I bleed to death having my period?" rounded out the anonymous pit of questions.

Puberty is an awakening of the ovaries from a dormant stage. Body fat is the major trigger for this awakening. The pituitary gland releases *luteinizing hormone* (LH), *growth hormone,* and FSH to create the physical changes of puberty: breast growth, a spurt in height, and underarm and pubic hair. Activity between the teen brain and hormone center can lead to acne, bloating, and breast tenderness or heavy bleeding and emotional hurricanes. Any parent of a young pubescent girl can readily relate to the chaotic wave of emotions, attitude, and physical upheaval.

The brain and hormone stability lead women into their reproductive years, a time when they feel their best unless premenstrual syndrome (PMS) challenges the system. Let's take a look at the normal hormone system, which resembles a thermostat. Just as the thermostat in your house turns off the heat when a heightened temperature is recognized, hormones signal each other, and the menstrual cycle, and ovulation, the peak time for conception.

To keep it simple, this discussion focuses on the major players involved in the menstrual cycle: estrogen, progesterone, FSH, and LH. Although most of us are led to believe that a 28-day cycle is the norm, research establishes that only 12.4 percent of women experience that time frame. Cycles can last anywhere between 24 and 35 days, with 20 percent of women experiencing irregular cycles.[4]

We will use a 28-day cycle for this account (see Figure 2.2). The first phase is the *follicular phase,* which extends from day 1 to day 14 and prepares the follicle (immature egg) for fertilization. Bleeding starts on day 1, and estrogen and progesterone are at their lowest levels. At this low level, the thermostat turns on and alerts the pituitary gland to begin producing FSH, which propels the follicles in the ovary to ripen. Testosterone remains fairly stable during the follicular phase and produces a sense of confidence, mental alertness, and sexual attunement. Follicles are eggs surrounded by a layer of hormone-producing cells. Although many follicles develop because of the introduction of FSH, only one, the dominate follicle, matures to ovulation. Follicles secrete estrogen, causing blood to advance to the uterine lining to prepare it for implantation of the egg. During the first 12 days of the cycle, FSH and estrogen levels are rising as the estrogen level reaches a set point; the thermostat signals the pituitary to stop producing FSH and to begin secreting LH. The LH surge causes the egg to be released from the ovary and travel down the fallopian tube for possible fertilization. This process is known as *ovulation,* which occurs at about day 14. Near ovulation, testosterone peaks slightly (as the brain is more efficient, providing a heightened sense of alertness), athletic skills peak, the sense of smell becomes more acute, and sexual desire increases.[5] The second phase of the menstrual cycle is called the *secretory phase,* which is responsible for secreting progesterone. The corpus luteum (empty follicle) secretes its own estrogen and progesterone. The uterine lining is matured by the hormone progesterone, preparing now for potential pregnancy. As progesterone establishes its high level, the thermostat is signaled by the pituitary to shut off the production of LH.

Both FSH and LH are shut off; however, the corpus luteum continues to pump out estrogen and progesterone until about day 22. If fertilization occurs, the fertilized egg secretes hormones to sustain itself. When fertilization does not occur, levels of progesterone and estrogen continue their decline. The rapid decline of these hormones occurs about five to seven days before menstruation begins and can produce premenstrual symptoms.

Blood vessels in the uterine wall, now void of estrogen and progesterone, begin to contract and spasm, causing the uterine lining to shed blood cells and mucous; monthly bleeding begins again. Low levels of estrogen and progesterone on day 1 ignite the thermostat, calling the pituitary gland back into service. The pituitary's tightly regulated system releasing FSH and LH bears a remarkable responsibility in the reproductive cycle.

Today, new freedom is offered to woman through use of hormonal contraception-like birth control pills. Women are choosing to limit menstrual cycles by artificially adjusting the estrogen-to-progesterone balance. These pills, patches, and vaginal rings release enough progesterone to prevent the brain from generating the LH signal, which releases the egg and inhibits vaginal bleeding by stabilizing any further growth of the uterine lining. Women find less bloating, irritability, and mood swings when utilizing these products

Figure 2.2
Menstrual Cycle

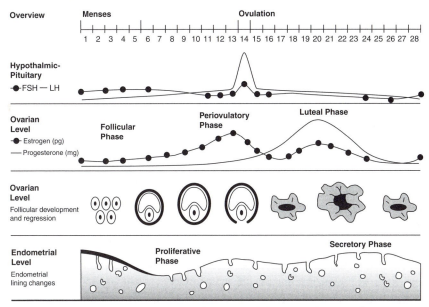

Source: Courtesy North American Menopause Society. North American Menopause Society, *Menopause Practice: A Clinician's Guide*, 3rd ed. (Cleveland, OH: North American Menopause Society, 2007), p. 20.

and are free from monthly periods. Hurray for chemical research and more options for women!

HORMONE HAPPENINGS

The onset of puberty and the menstrual cycle, which is responsible for establishing a fertile reproductive environment, is highly orchestrated by hormone production. Hormones continue their strategic role as women transition from the reproductive to the postreproductive years. Fertility rates begin their descent about the mid-thirties, leaving hormonal regulation in a chaotic and unpredictable state, while at the same time a wild ride ensues of heavy bleeding one month and scant bleeding the next month, hot flashes, insomnia, mood swings, and irritability. The culprits of this chaotic period of life are once again hormones. Hormones are the chemicals secreted by various glands and tissues in the body that then circulate in the blood to control the function of certain cells and organs. The brain is the master control agent and seeks to maintain a balance of hormones produced, those circulating in the bloodstream, and the interrelationship of these messengers for the body's state of well-being. Over the past 10 years, many new hormones have been discovered, and research continues to uncover more; more than 200 are known today.[6] Without the work of hormones in your body temperature regulation, sleep, thirst, hunger, and sex would malfunction.

Endocrine System

The hypothalamus is the interpretation and processing center for hormones; in addition, this master signaler sends out hormonal messages to the rest of the body, ultimately controlling body temperature, blood pressure, sleep, hunger, thirst, sleep, arousal, and emotions.

The nine endocrine glands that produce hormones are the thyroid, parathyroid, pituitary, pineal, pancreas, adrenals (two), gonads-ovaries (two), and testes (two). However, hormones are also released by skin, bone, white blood cells, the stomach, and fat, or adipose, tissue. They have a unique relay system that acts to maintain a balance with four major hormone systems: sex hormones, metabolic hormones, regulatory hormones, and stress hormones. The major system for our purpose is the *sex hormone system*. Estrogen, progesterone, and testosterone are the major players. They are produced mainly by the ovaries, adrenal glands, and body fat, and these marvelous messengers can be converted into one another by enzymes and feedback loops. There is a complex interaction between the hypothalamus, pituitary gland, and ovaries that promotes their primary role in reproduction. Secondarily, they influence mood, temperature, appetite, and sleep.

Let us take a closer look at the impact of perimenopause on the sex hormones. As early perimenopause ushers in, the ovaries produce less estrogen, and the brain tries to compensate for the decrease in estrogen by sending more FSH. As FSH rises, the ovaries recruit more than the traditional dozen follicles to produce estrogen for the next menstrual cycle. Periods become more erratic, the length of the cycle shifts by seven or more days from its norm, one or two cycles in a row are missed, and intervals between periods lengthen until menstruation stops. The elevation of FSH is a hallmark of reproductive aging. An accelerated loss of follicles contributes to an increasing level of FSH. The marked increase is apparent at least two years before the FMP and then plateaus within two years after FMP. These FSH findings assist clinicians in assessing the phase of a woman's reproductive aging.

Estrogen

Estrogen has received a significant amount of research since the 1950s with the publication of *Forever Young*, a book extolling the benefits of estrogen to promote antiaging in women. Studies actually reveal that most U.S. women are experiencing symptoms of either estrogen excess or progesterone defiency.[7] During puberty, estrogen is responsible for the development of pubic hair and breasts and the development of the uterus for menstruation. In women during the reproductive age, the ovary is the major source of estrogen. Estrogen's basic functions are regrowing uterine lining, maintaining vaginal and bladder tissue health, decreasing bone loss, stimulating breast cells, and sustaining mood, cognition, and concentration. Women produce three types of estrogen: *estrone* (E1), *estradiol* (E2), and *estriol* (E3).

Estrone (E1) is produced primarily by the ovaries prior to perimenopause. Postmenopause, it is produced by conversion of androgens in fat stores. Some refer to estrone as the "bad" estrogen. In normal quantities, it is relatively harmless; in large amounts, it challenges the work of estradiol and is associated with an increased risk of breast cancer. Estrone's major value is that it can be converted into estradiol.

Estradiol (E2) is the strongest estrogen but is produced in the smallest amounts of all the sex hormones. Estradiol is made by the ovaries and the one most people are referring to when discussing estrogen. It has more than 300 functions in the body, including promoting neuron growth, hardening bones, dilating blood vessels, promoting sexual lubrication, causing positive mood changes and normal sleep cycles, and maintaining balance, coordination, smell, hearing, and skin tone. No wonder that as estrogen fades, many normal body functions slip and that those disruptive symptoms, such as hot flashes, insomnia, and irritability, take over. Fat tissue is another source of estrogen production and possibly the main source for obese women in menopause transition. One vitally important major function to the aging woman is that estradiol slows brain aging by stimulating nerve growth, function, and healing.

Estriol (E3) is the weakest of the three estrogens. Pregnancy is the only time it is produced in excess amounts. It promotes blood flow to the uterus during pregnancy and helps an expecting mother get rid of unneeded hormones produced by the fetus.

Phytoestrogens are weak plant estrogens. The most studied phytoestrogen is soy. Plants and animals produce hormones that behave like human hormones. They can bind to estrogen receptors in the cell and provide adequate stimulation to cells for estrogen-deficient women. *Xenoestrogens* are the most potent estrogens. They are not found in the human body, in animals, or in plants but are by-products of commercial compounds, such as petrochemical-based plastics, medicines, clothing, cleansers, and pesticides. Many pesticides and organic solvents behave like estrogens when consumed or absorbed by the human body. Alone or in small quantities, they are not harmful. However, when combined with multiple xenoestrogens, they have a synergistic effect and can be harmful to humans. The pesticide DDT was banned because of its harmful effects more than 25 years ago, yet it can remain active in the soil for more than 25 years, affecting food products. And what about the countries we import food from that do not ban DDT?

Excess Estrogen Can Cause or Worsen the Following

- Irregular/heavy bleeding
- Breast tenderness
- Depression, fatigue, and poor concentration
- Fibrocystic breast
- PMS
- Decreased libido
- Fibroid growth
- Endometriosis
- Water retention and bloating
- Fat gain around the hips and thighs
- Breast and uterine cancer

Estrogen Deficiency Can Cause or Worsen the Following

- Vaginal dryness
- Decreased sex drive
- Disturbed sleep
- Poor concentration
- Depression
- Thinning skin[8]

Progesterone

Progesterone, a sex steroid hormone, is produced by the corpus luteum only after ovulation. Its main function is to promote and maintain pregnancy. Another function is to regulate estrogen activity. Progesterone is a precursor of estrogen and testosterone, and it is the first hormone to decline in perimenopause. Progestins are compounds similar to progesterone in chemical makeup and are often used to treat vaginal bleeding. When ovulation ceases, progesterone is not produced; then the only defense against excess estrogen in the body is androgen metabolism. Ultimately, it is the healthy balance of estrogen and progesterone that helps women function at their best.

Functions of Progesterone

- Necessary for the survival of embryo and fetus
- Protects against fibrocystic breasts
- A natural diuretic, decreasing water retention
- Natural antidepressant and antianxiety hormone
- Restores sex drive
- Builds bone
- Decreases uterine contractions (cramping)
- Decreases frequency of seizures

Hormone balance is important. Without the proper concentration and ratio of hormones to one another, optimal function is altered and will affect many body systems, ultimately creating an illness. Estrogen and progesterone have a ratio to maintain: 20 to 1 after ovulation (ratio of free estrogen to free progesterone). This simple statistic becomes the heart of the story for the perimenopausal woman whose estrogen is declining, while at the same time the end of ovulation renders progesterone at its lowest level. The further disruption of hormone balance for U.S. women relates to lifestyle, diet, exposure to external estrogens, delayed childbirth, and the extreme stress that so many women face. Asian women with a traditional Asian diet have minimal menopausal symptoms, breast cancer, PMS, and fibroids—that is, until they are Americanized by living in the larger cities or moving to the United States. I have faith in the awareness and commitment of American women to alter their lifestyles, thus improving life in their menopause years. But it will mean low-fat, high-fiber diets with at least four servings of fruit and vegetables a day; exercise to minimize a sedentary existence; and reduction of demanding roles, expectations, and stress levels.

Testosterone

Testosterone is not just a male hormone; its primary job for males and females is to provide energy and sex drive, stimulate muscle growth, and help you burn calories. This androgen, unlike estrogen and progesterone, does not seek a balance or ratio; it is produced in equal amounts until menopause. Your adrenal glands and ovaries produce most of the androgens in your body with a smaller amount converted by skin and muscle. A man's body produces 20 times more testosterone than a woman's. After a woman's twentieth birthday, testosterone levels decrease every year; at age 40, the production is only half the amount at age 20 and will continue to decline by 90 percent at late menopause. A fact unknown by most, as testosterone declines in menopause, the metabolism declines, and fat deposits build. For some, building up the testosterone stores can help decrease the weight gain that is so troublesome to women in menopause and help restore some libido. Even though the debate continues regarding testosterone therapy, it can be combined with estrogen to increase metabolism, sexual function, and well-being. Dr. Susan Davis, professor of women's health in Prahran, Australia, has led recent clinical trials to determine the health risks and benefits of testosterone therapy. I heard her presentation at the 2007 North American Menopause Society Conference, and she is indeed a champion for women's health and hormone options.

What will the next generation say of menopause? If today is an indicator, women of the next decade, with their technologic savvy, demanding voices, and sense of entitlement, will be breaking through more than a glass ceiling. Their insistence on voicing their health concerns, the rich research they will bring to a provider, along with their own individualized health plan can leave little of today's conservative models intact. And you, the mothers, grandmothers, teachers, and mentors of these fine women, have set the stage and shared your knowledge of the critical need for hormone balance throughout life; modeled a healthy lifestyle with exercise, diet, and stress reduction; and even taken it one step further—you are the revitalized seasoned women, physically, emotionally, and sexually.

Chapter Three

THE CHANGING BODY OF THE PERIMENOPAUSAL AND MENOPAUSAL WOMAN

Time is a dressmaker, specializing in alterations.

—Faith Baldwin

Debbie was 47 years old when she first came to the office. She sat in the waiting room waving a brochure to fan herself while she filled out her demographic information. Debbie looked up at me with those pleading eyes and said, "I hope you can help me. I just cannot live like this!" Her story sounded too familiar. She had a hysterectomy at age 43 for abnormal uterine bleeding and fibroids. Debbie described her relief to no longer have that monthly outpouring. Then the hot flashes started with the nights of little sleep. Her family practice physician put her on Estratest. After eight months of hormone therapy (HT) and without relief of her symptoms, she took herself off the medication. Two years later, Debbie was no better, and the hot flashes had invaded her days, not just the nights. I saw her about a year postmeds, and the picture was even more charged. Her sleep cycle was disrupted to the point of waking every two hours, drenched in perspiration, and her level of irritability affected her relationship with her husband and daughters. She told me I was her last resort—not a great place to find yourself as a clinician. Could I help her? At the very least, I could begin an assessment process, do saliva testing of her sex hormones and adrenals, and be a support as we unraveled her options.

Debbie had adrenal fatigue with a midnight cortisol level almost off the charts. Her estrogen was a little low for her age and hormone state, but her progesterone was very low. That would account for her severe vasomotor symptoms (hot flashes and night sweats). We started HT with Combi patch (estrdiol/norethindrone acetate transdermal system). Two weeks after treatment, Debbie returned for follow-up, saying, "Dona, I cannot believe it. I haven't had any hot flashes during the day. After that first day I put on the patch, and only one hot flash at night and no sweating. My husband and I can cuddle at night like we use to when we fell asleep. My friends can even tell that I am better. I could just hug you! You have to tell other women, there is help, they do not have to suffer through menopause!"

I am trying to inform other women that they do not have to suffer forever with the various menopause-related symptoms. Talk to your health care provider, share your story, and discuss your testing options to determine a hormone baseline (whether serum/blood or saliva) and what treatment options are available. If your provider is not approachable, find another one who is. Do not assume that every physician has a working knowledge of women's health issues and of menopause in particular. Just like every nurse is not a nurse, each health professional has a general knowledge of health care, and most specialize in a particular field of interest or several. It is ridiculous to expect your provider to know everything about all facets of the human body. My recommendation is that you find a clinician who does have an expertise in women's health and share your needs. Chapter 4 gives more specifics to prepare you to interview the provider. Remember that it is *your* health and well-being.

Debbie's story presents a postmenopausal woman some four years after hysterectomy. What about the perimenopausal woman in early stages who is aggravated by symptoms but not so severe that she is ready to try HT? Disruptive menopausal symptoms affect approximately 70 percent of perimenopausal women, with 20 percent less bothered by hormone fluctuations and 10 percent who can find themselves incapacitated like Debbie.[1] This chapter outlines the changing body of the perimenopausal and menopausal woman. Common concerns appear from irregular uterine bleeding, vasomotor symptoms, sleep disturbances, cognitive changes, sexual changes, pelvic pain, weight gain, and cardiovascular disease. Whether you ever experience issues beyond the temporary annoyance of hot flashes and insomnia, women need to know the potential changes to their bodies and be alert to the early warning signals of disease processes such as hypertension, diabetes, and heart disease. I believe that *knowledge is power*. Be a powerful health care consumer and help prepare those young women—your daughters, nieces, and granddaughters—in the next generation.

PERIMENOPAUSE: THE BEGINNING

Evelyn is 36 years old and has been married for 10 years. She and her husband have a two-year-old son. Recently, she has noticed irregular, heavy bleeding as well as additional cramping and more moodiness. Perimenopause can occur from approximately 30 to 45 years old, the menstrual cycle becomes irregular because ovulation is erratic due to hormone fluctuations. These fluctuations and the symptoms that follow can last anywhere from 1 to 15 years. If ovulation does not occur and progesterone is not produced, the menstrual cycle becomes uncertain, and instead of the next month's cycle occurring 14 days after ovulation, the time shifts. A woman's peak time for reproduction is between ages 18 and 35; ovulation, the timekeeper of the menstrual cycle, remains steady. Then one month ovulation does not occur (anovulation), and estrogen is produced without the needed amount of progesterone to sustain hormone balance. The uterine lining is thicker, the uterus does not know it is time to shed the lining since ovulation did not occur, and the heavy and erratic menstrual cycles begin.

Fertility declines significantly in women around age 35 to 38. In fact, the ovary contains the maximum number of cells that mature into eggs during a woman's fetal development. Women are born with 1 million to 2 million follicles, and by menopause only a few hundred to a few thousand remain. At approximately age 37, follicles decline steeply in number and stability.[2] As the eggs age and ovulation becomes erratic, a wide range of problems can occur for women: pregnancy is more difficult, birth defects are more frequent, fibroids appear, menstrual cycles are irregular, the risk of breast cancer increases, bone loss begins, weight increases, and emotions are more chaotic. Pregnancy is more difficult, but a word of caution for the perimenopausal woman: pregnancy is still possible until menopause (no menstrual period for 12 consecutive months). Perimenopausal women have a range of *contraception* options to explore, including the most drastic sterilization (tubal ligation and vasectomy), barrier methods (spermicides, condoms, diaphragms, cervical caps, and cervical sponges), hormonal contraceptives, and intrauterine devices. The point is to protect yourself from an unwanted pregnancy and do not be lulled into believing that pregnancy won't happen to you.

Additional complaints are voiced by Evelyn. She has less energy, more food cravings, and bloating, and her breasts are tender. Since she is not ovulating efficiently, her body is producing more estrogen than progesterone; this can affect her thyroid hormone production, slowing down metabolism and the body's ability to process food into energy. Evelyn is frustrated by this latest development. She claims to eat a balanced diet, exercises regularly, and sleeps a fair amount but still has little energy, and the weight gain seems to tip her mood into irritability. The bloating, breast tenderness, and swelling of her hands and feet are the result of a progesterone deficiency and the absence of its diuretic effect. Estrogen is continuing its production, but progesterone cannot keep up without ovulation. These lower levels of progesterone affect her concentration, her mood, and possibly her sex drive since progesterone is needed to produce testosterone, which stimulates libido in women.

Any one of these complaints could frustrate Evelyn, but the cascade of changes and her determination to make wise choices for herself and increase her understanding of what is happening to her body will be one reason she buys a book like this and reads this chapter. One-third of all American women are now between ages 40 and 60, some 37 million strong, and they are somewhere in the menopause transition attempting to understand it, unravel its impact on their lives, and be informed to negotiate their way through midlife successfully.[3] These educated women realize that by making wise choices during their transition, they can live longer, be healthier, and enter their second adulthood with the vitality to accomplish the list of things they now have time to invest in.

CHANGES IN UTERINE BLEEDING

Approximately 90 percent of women experience some form of change in their menstrual cycle during the four- to eight-year period before the onset of menopause. Changes in the flow and frequency of menses are the hallmarks of perimenopause.[4] The majority of women hardly notice the subtle changes of perimenopause, such as lighter bleeding, heavier bleeding, bleeding that lasts less than two days or greater than four days, cycle length of less than seven days or greater than 28 days, or perhaps a skipped menstrual period. All this can represent an array of consequences for women: avoiding sexual activities, heavy or prolonged bleeding that can produce social embarrassment or even anemia, and a diminished quality of life.

Since changes in uterine bleeding may be a signal of illness or a disease process of the reproductive system, women are encouraged to keep good records of the changes and discuss the changes with their providers at annual exams or make an earlier appointment. In the perimenopausal woman, the cause is the generally erratic ovulation process that creates an imbalance of estrogen and progesterone. However, since anything from infection, thyroid changes, polycystic ovarian syndrome, fibroids, cancer, and even leukemia can be the culprit, a perimenopausal woman who is not using any type of oral HT should have a history taken and a pelvic exam. The age of a woman and her stage of menopause often determine how extensive an evaluation is needed.

A few important points need to be made regarding women who start bleeding only after initiation of estrogen/progesterone therapy (EPT). If the bleeding is not heavy and declines over time, it needs no evaluation. A perimenopausal or menopausal woman using EPT whose uterine bleeding persists longer than six months or longer than one week each month in the first six months of therapy should be evaluated to rule out a bigger problem. The TREMIN Research Program on Women's Health (the oldest ongoing study of menstruation in the country, now based at Penn State University) reports that 4 out of 100 women do have menstrual cycles after their final menstrual period. Periods may be triggered from stress or other environmental issues. An anecdotal story was shared with me from a woman in her twenties. Her mother had been on Depo-Provera injections for years that led to six years of no menstrual cycles; two years ago, she stopped the injections and remained period free. "My mother just had a period. She is 58 years old and was shocked after all these years that her cycle returned. This past week she has not been herself—irritable, withdrawn, she won't leave the house. She says she feels like an adolescent just having her first period." Women who have been on oral contraceptives into those years of transition (thirties to fifties) are encouraged by most physicians to stop taking the pill, at least for a trial, around age 51 to see whether they have reached menopause and no longer need to be on higher levels of hormones required for contraception. Letting your body find its balance and determining your transition into natural menopause is your decision and ultimately your journey.

MANAGEMENT OF ABNORMAL UTERINE BLEEDING

The change in menstrual bleeding is one of the primary symptoms alerting a woman to the onset of perimenopause. When the irregular bleeding is excessive or erratic, it is generally from a benign or malignant cause and requires evaluation. Management of abnormal uterine bleeding (AUB) in perimenopausal and menopausal women covers a wide range of effective options, both medical and surgical. Hormonal options include combination estrogen-progestin oral contraceptives, transdermal and vaginal ring contraceptives, continuous injectable or intrauterine progestin contraceptives, oral EPT, cyclic oral progestogen alone, and intravenous estrogen for emergency situations. Estrogen-containing contraception is not recommended for women with a history of deep-vein thrombosis (blood clots) or other cardiovascular risks or women over age 35 who smoke.

Several surgical options to treat women with AUB are *dilation and curettage* (D&C) with hysteroscopy, endometrial ablation, and hysterectomy. For two reasons, D&C is now considered obsolete to treat AUB. First, with this blind procedure, a clinician can miss a local disease, such as polyps, and, second, not all the tissue can be removed.[5] With hysteroscopy, D&C is effective in making diagnoses. One safe and cost-effective alternative to hysterectomy for treatment of AUB is *endometrial resection and ablation.*

Endometrial ablation is an outpatient surgical procedure often taking from 15 to 45 minutes, meaning that after recovery from anesthesia, a woman usually goes home the same day. This procedure is used to treat heavy or prolonged menstrual bleeding when bleeding has not responded to other treatments, childbearing is complete, other medical problems prevent hysterectomy, or a hysterectomy is not desired. Endometrial ablation uses a lighted viewing instrument (hysteroscope) and other instruments to destroy (ablate) the uterine lining or endometrium. The procedure can be done by laser beam, freezing, electricity, or heat (thermal ablation) using radiofrequency or a balloon filled with heated saline solution. Approximately 90 percent of women will have reduced menstrual flow, and up to half will stop having periods after ablation.[6]

In 2005, there were 617,000 *hysterectomies* performed in the United States. According to the National Center for Health Statistics, of the 617,000 hysterectomies performed in 2004, 73 percent also involved the surgical removal of the ovaries. In the United States, one-third of women can be expected to have a hysterectomy by age 60. Currently, there are an estimated 22 million women in the United States who have undergone this procedure; that is an average of 622,000 hysterectomies a year over the past decade with an average cost of approximately $5 billion a year.[7] The first hysterectomy was performed in 1843 by Charles Clay in Manchester, England, and in 1929, Dr. Edward Richardson performed the first total abdominal hysterectomy.[8]

Hysterectomy is the surgical removal of the uterus. A total hysterectomy removes the entire uterus, including the cervix. Subtotal hysterectomy removes only the upper body of the uterus, leaving the cervix in place. Oophorectomy is the surgical removal of the ovary, and salpingo-oophorectomy is the removal of the ovary and fallopian tube. Removal of a woman's uterus leaves her unable to bear children and changes the hormonal levels considerably; thus, surgery is recommended only when necessary for the following conditions: treatment of uterine, cervical, and ovarian cancer; severe and intractable endometriosis; vaginal prolapse; heavy or uncontrolled menstrual bleeding; postpartum for severe placenta praevia; as a last resort with excessive postpartum bleeding; and a prophylactic treatment for those with a strong family history of reproductive system cancers. For decades, women experienced hysterectomy with removal of both ovaries. Today, physicians recognize the need to leave one or both ovaries to supplement estrogen sources as a woman ages. The ovaries continue to produce lower levels of estrogen for the postmenopausal woman; additional estrogen comes from body fat and other smaller sources in the body.

Although hysterectomy is frequently performed for *fibroids* (benign tumor-like growths inside the uterus), conservative treatment options are available. Myomectomy is surgical removal of fibroids that leaves the uterus intact and has been performed for more than a century. Fibroids account for one-third of hysterectomies and one-fifth of gynecological visits. *Endometriosis* is responsible for approximately one-fifth of hysterectomies, and it affects women during their reproductive years. It is a disease in which tissue similar to the endometrium (lining of the uterus) is present outside the uterus in other parts of the body. Scar tissue can form in the areas of endometriosis—bladder, intestines, bowel, colon, and rectum—creating severe pelvic pain, infertility, and miscarriages. The most common gynecological cancer in the United States is cancer of the uterus, with an estimated 36,100 new cases in 2000, affecting women ages 35 to 90 with a mean age of 62 years. This invasive cancer may originate in the endometrium and spread to other reproductive organs or the rest of the body.[9]

The hysterectomy procedure is surrounded by controversy. It is the second most common major operation performed in the United States today, second only to cesarean section. Other countries, such as England, Sweden, and France, have up to four times fewer hysterectomies performed annually. The decision to have a hysterectomy should not be taken lightly. New technology, new medical treatments, and new gynecological procedures to treat severe pain and bleeding are being discovered. Ultimately, the decision is yours; the most important factor in helping you choose appropriate medical care is your comprehensive understanding of the reasons for treatment, the risks, and the potential benefits. And a second opinion before proceeding to major surgery that is life altering is always your option.

VASOMOTOR SYMPTOMS

Vasomotor sensations that range from warmth to intense heat in the upper body and face and can be followed by chills are known as *hot flashes*. The intense perspiration while sleeping is called *night sweats*. The hot flash is the second most frequently reported perimenopausal symptom and can last one to five minutes. It is believed that they may result from the estrogen and progesterone fluctuations during menopause transition. If fact, studies continue to unearth the cause of the dreaded hot flash; until recently, the hypothalamus was believed to set hot flashes in motion. It has also been postulated that the unnatural estrogenic substances caused by pollutants in the environment, the xenoestrogens, may be precipitating "ovarian dysfunction," perhaps a reason that more women in industrialized countries experience hot flashes than women in Third World countries. Research continues, and women globally await the news of what causes a hot flash so that an effective treatment can be proposed.

A few substantive studies are highlighted to demonstrate the frequency of hot flashes in this time of transition. The North American Menopause Society (NAMS) chronicled a 2007 systematic review of papers addressing the worldwide prevalence of hot flashes; 41 percent of perimenopausal women and 41.5 percent of postmenopausal women reported this menacing symptom.[10] The Study of Women's Health Across the Nation evaluated a multiracial and multiethnic sample of 16,065 women aged 40 to 55 and concluded that African American women have the most frequent symptoms (45.6%) followed by Hispanic (35.4%), white (31.2%), Chinese (20.5%), and Japanese (17.6%) women.[11] Researchers and clinicians alike believe that a more important indicator of having hot flashes is body mass index. Discussion of lifestyle changes and healthy living to combat hot flashes appears later in this section.

Knowing that some 75 percent of perimenopausal women in the United States claim hot flashes as a bothersome life challenge and an acute discomfort leading to loss of sleep and greatly impacting the quality of life, it becomes imperative that the cause and treatment be identified. I see too many women, partners, children, colleagues, and friends waiting in anticipation of this resolution. We also know that hot flashes can continue 10 years or longer for a woman, with the most common cases revealing hot flashes lasting between two months and two years. Postmenopausal women have an increased risk of hot flashes during the first two years of their final menstrual period that can decline overtime. Hot flashes seem to be influenced by climate, diet, lifestyle, a woman's role, and her attitude regarding the end of fertility and her aging process. Women with surgically induced menopause often have more severe hot flashes. Sufferers of premenstrual syndrome with severe symptoms during their reproductive years claim an incidence of intense hot flashes in perimenopause of 47 percent versus 32 percent of women without a history of severe premenstrual syndrome.[12] I do see this connection in clinical practice. These women are often the ones who fall in that 10 percent with severe menopausal symptoms who often fail bioidenticals and need a stronger treatment or even several interventions after lifestyle changes have not improved their wellbeing. Dr. Robert Greene raises the question of nerve damage to the brain during hot flashes and concern for women in their later years with conditions like Alzheimer's disease. His early studies found that blood flow to the brain decreases dramatically during a hot flash, especially in the regions of the brain responsible for verbal memory and short-term memory.[13]

That makes perfect sense to me. I have been honored with the North Carolina Nurses Association's Board of Directors Award for Outstanding Service. I was very surprised and caught off guard; as I was walking to the podium, I experienced an intense hot flash. My face was dark red, I could feel the perspiration at my scalp, and by the time I reached the front of the room, I was short of breath and could not think of a thing to say. My verbal skills were in my feet; how many brain cells did I lose with that one?

MANAGEMENT OF HOT FLASHES

More than 25 percent of women have significant discomfort and loss of quality of life from hot flashes, thus sending them to health care providers to request information and treatment. Women describe sensations of their skin crawling, heart palpitations, faintness, and enveloping heat rising from their midchest to the hair follicles. There is no cure for these flashes, and offering symptom relief is often the best a clinician can do.[14] For a smaller number of women, the frequency of hot flashes will often stop without treatment. If you have been one of those women with severe flashes, you know that waiting for them to stop after about two months of significant discomfort is just not an option. Take heart; my message is this: do not delay if you have severe symptoms—get the intervention you need and do not jeopardize your quality of life.

Before treatment, prepare a detailed history of the frequency and severity of hot flashes and the effects on your daily life. If they are not bothersome, do not treat them. This is where a Hot Flash Diary, noting the date, time of day, activity during hot flash, intensity, and any intervention you attempted, is very helpful. My clients come in with pages of incidents over a two-week period. This information makes treatment so much easier.

2004 NAMS Suggested Options for Women with Vasomotor Symptoms

- Enhance relaxation with meditation, yoga, massage, or a leisurely lukewarm bath
- Get regular exercise to promote better, more restorative sleep
- Keep cool by dressing in layers, using a fan, and sleeping in a cool room
- Maintain a healthy body weight
- Do not smoke
- When a hot flash starts, try using paced respiration (deep, slow, abdominal breathing)
- Avoid perceived hot flash triggers (hot drinks, caffeine, spicy foods, and alcohol), although studies to date do not support the association
- Try nonprescription therapies (soy foods/isoflavones, black cohosh, or vitamin E) for mild hot flashes, although evidence is mixed
- For moderate to severe hot flashes, consider HT (the only government-approved treatment) or nonestrogen prescription drugs (progestogens, transdermal clonidine, venlafaxine, or gabapentin)[15]

Lifestyle changes remain the first line of intervention for women with mild hot flashes. Clinicians report frequent stories from women suggesting a relationship between the severity of hot flashes and emotional stress. Paying attention to triggers of your stress may help you bypass a hot flash. Keep a reasonable schedule during times when the flashes are pronounced. Again, for many women, they do not last forever but can have peak periods during your transition. Keep up the yoga, meditation, walks after dinner, and exercise to promote balance in your life. A new study from the University of California, San Francisco, hints that taking weekly yoga classes may cut a woman's number of hot flashes each week by 30 percent. Another way to decrease the severity of nighttime hot flashes is through seven weeks of acupuncture. A Stanford University study notes a 28 percent decrease compared to a 6 percent decrease for a sham treatment. The important point is to work with a licensed acupuncturist who treats hot flashes.[16] One report showed that women who engaged in at least 40 minutes of aerobic exercise three times a week reduced their hot flashes by about 50 percent compared to a sedentary group.[17]

Walk through any store these days and notice the seasoned women dressed in layers with a light jacket thrown over an arm, a note card in her hand fanning herself, and beads of perspiration on her upper lip or forehead. I can certainly relate to dressing in layers. Recommending "menopause survival kits for hot flashes" is another empathetic connection. Besides dressing in layers, I encourage women to keep a small bag in their desk drawer or trunk of the car containing a plastic bag for dampened clothing, a dry bra, a dry white cotton shirt (that can go with about everything), deodorant, perfume, a facecloth or small towel, and moist towelettes. Sleeping in a cool room at night is one option; recently, I was introduced to a new silk-like bedding fabric (Derma-Therapy) made from patented fabrics that wick moisture from the skin. These pillow cases and sheets have made many of my clients lives better during the provoking sleep periods with night sweats. Information for Cool Sets, Derma-Therapy, and Wild Bleu is available for women wanting to sleep with less distress.[18]

If after lifestyle changes you have not received adequate relief, you may want to explore nonprescription remedies, prescription therapies, and hormone options. These modalities are outlined in chapter 4. Decisions about HT are between you and your health care provider. Any decision you make is not final and should be reviewed annually at your checkup.

SLEEP DISTURBANCES

A National Sleep Foundation survey in 2007 notes about 46 percent of U.S. women aged 40 to 54 and 48 percent aged 55 to 64 report sleep problems. Various factors can account for sleep disturbances with this population in addition to the hormonal changes and stress-significant life challenges, such as loss of life partners through death or divorce, care of elderly or young family members, job-related stress, and chronic illness. Further, the survey revealed that peri- and postmenopausal women sleep less, have more frequent insomnia symptoms, and are more than twice as likely to use prescription sleeping aids as premenopausal women. The majority of people do not voluntarily report sleep disturbances to clinicians, nor do most clinicians ask about them. If adequate sleep for most adults is approximately six to nine hours per night and allows them to function in an alert state during waking hours, then *poor sleep*, a subjective assessment, is an inadequate quantity or poor quality of sleep. Poor sleep is associated with tension, irritability, fatigue, lethargy, inability to concentrate, lack of motivation, and difficulty performing tasks. It has also been linked to chronic illness, cardiac problems, depression, and mood disorders. Negative outcomes from poor sleep are increased automobile accidents and work-related injuries.[19] The last two issues alone are a reason that clinicians need to be vigilant in asking about sleep problems and consumers need to share this vital information.

An individual with *insomnia* can complain of several issues related to their poor quality of sleep: difficultly falling asleep, waking up frequently during the night with difficulty returning to sleep, waking up too early in the morning, and unrefreshing sleep. It is defined less by the number of hours of sleep. There are at least three types of insomnia: transient, acute, and chronic. *Transient insomnia* lasts from days to weeks and can be caused by other disorders, by changes in the sleep environment and the timing of sleep, or by stress. *Acute insomnia* is the inability to consistently sleep well for a period of between three weeks and six months. *Chronic insomnia* lasts from months to years and can also be caused by sleep-disordered breathing, such as sleep apnea and other disorders. A referral to a sleep center to evaluate sleep apnea, restless legs syndrome, narcolepsy (uncontrollable sleep bouts during waking hours), excessive daytime sleepiness, upper airway dynamics, hormonal influences, and weight issues is always warranted for ongoing sleep disruption.

MANAGEMENT OF SLEEP DISTURBANCES

Clinicians should ask each peri- and postmenopausal woman about her quality of sleep. Can you get to sleep? Do you have early morning awakening? Do you feel rested on awakening? But if your health care provider doesn't ask, by all means tell him or her about the quality of your sleep. Treatment for sleep disorders can be behavioral or prescriptive. There are a few basics of "sleep hygiene" to promote sleep for the peri- and postmenopausal woman. First, avoid caffeine, chocolate, cola drinks, alcohol, and nicotine close to bedtime. Some use alcohol to relax, but if you are having sleep disturbances, alcohol can have a rebound effect, giving you fragmented sleep and early awakening. It also tends to swell the nasal mucosa, worsening snoring, and for those with sleep apnea, matters become worse. Try not to watch intense, action-packed television an hour before sleep, as it has a tendency to get the heart racing and is not conducive to winding down before sleep. Establishing sleep hygiene or nightly rituals is a benefit: a cool, quiet, dark room and reserving the bedroom for sleep only, not work. If you are not asleep after 15 minutes of awakening, get up, read, watch television, do relaxation exercises, or go to another room to sleep. And a regular sleep schedule, even on weekends, to promote synchrony will help restore the quality of sleep. Weight loss and moderate exercise to decrease the body mass index (BMI) and promote sleep are the mainstays for healthy sleep patterns. Nasal continuous positive airway pressure (CPAP) remains the standard of apnea treatment, although some women appear to have difficulty accepting this.

NONPRESCRIPTION AND PRESCRIPTION REMEDIES

Sleep cycle disruption and insomnia are common complaints in this fast-paced, jet-setting world. Often the first lines of treatment options are sedative or hypnotics to help people sleep; however, they have adverse effects, such as dependency, withdrawal symptoms, and rebound insomnia with lower doses. Botanical sedatives and *melatonin* can improve sleep without the adverse affects. *Valerian* is made from the roots of the valerian plant. It is used primarily to treat nervousness and insomnia and is recognized by the German health authorities and the World Health Organization for these purposes. Valerian improves the subjective experience of sleep when taken nightly for one to two weeks and is safe for mild to moderate insomnia at the usual dose of valerian extract 100 to 1,800 mg.[20]

Although there are few scientific studies, anecdotal reports of improved sleep exist for use of German chamomile, lavender, hop, lemon balm, and passion flower. Melatonin is a naturally occurring hormone that is secreted by the pineal gland to induce and maintain sleep. Melatonin production declines with age; some evidence shows that replacement may improve sleep efficiency and reduce awakenings. Doses range from 0.3 to 5 mg at bedtime; when taken for jet lag, doses of less than 4 mg are suggested. Melatonin should be taken for short duration up to two months. It should not be taken with drugs that supplement antiplatelet or anticoagulant properties because of its anticoagulant effect. It can produce excess sedation if taken with alcohol or Valium and Xanax.[21]

Sleeping pills (sedatives and hypnotics) may be used to break a cycle of insomnia but preferably as a last resort. Short-acting sleeping aids (Ambien with a four- to five-hour duration, Sonata with a one- to three-hour duration, and Lunesta with a six-hour duration) may be prescribed to promote sleep. They show fewer side effects like dependency and fewer withdrawal effects compared with benzodiazepines. Benzodiazepines, such as Valium and Xanax, have side effects, such as next-day sedation and dependence, and should be used at most a maximum of three nights per week. Rozerem assists with falling asleep. Trazodone, an antidepressant, is often prescribed off label as a sleep aid at a low dose of 25 to 50 mg at bedtime.[22]

Although HT has not been approved for treatment of insomnia, oral EPT has shown to improve nighttime restlessness and awakening and to reduce hot flashes and night sweats.

HEADACHES

Headaches are one of the most common problems reported in primary care settings. Headaches occurring more than twice a week should be charted and monitored and preventive medication considered. Many women can find headaches to be debilitating and frustrating and interfere with quality of life. There are three types of headaches: tension, cluster, and migraine. Data to record for proper diagnosis include the time the headache was experienced, symptoms, and potential triggers (stress, particular foods consumed, and menses). Causes of headaches range from infection, dental problems, allergies, colds, stress, environmental changes, and hormones for menopause and contraception, especially progestins. There is a clear connection between headaches and menstrual periods (menstrual migraines). Hormone therapy has been found to increase migraines in some women while easing them in others. Women experiencing migraines with auras should use great caution with hormone treatment because of an increased risk of stroke. Anne Mac-Gregor, MFFP, spoke at the 2007 NAMS conference, sharing her findings on hormones and headaches. Migraines increase during perimenopause and peak on or between two days before the start of menstruation and the first three days of bleeding. The good news is that menstrual migraines improve in postmenopause. Her suggestion for women with migraines either with or without aura is continuous transdermal estrogen in the lowest effective dose to prevent the "withdrawal" of estrogen. Headaches can be debilitating; a woman with headaches is best helped with a supportive relationship with her provider and good data to support her concerns (headache diary).

OTHER BODY CHANGES IN THE MENOPAUSE TRANSITION

Difficulty concentrating and remembering are common complaints during the menopause transition and early postmenopause. Sleep cycle changes, hot flashes, and various midlife changes may contribute to memory decline. There is no firm evidence that memory or other cognitive skills decline during natural menopause. Some women may encounter these problems, which are related more to aging than to menopause. Rapid transition into menopause with surgical menopause may have an effect on cognitive performance. Another component of cognitive function for the perimenopausal woman is mood changes, which have been observed in up to 10 percent of perimenopausal women participating in community-based studies. The most predictive factor for depression during midlife and beyond is a prior history of depression.[23] Vaginal changes also occur during midlife. Women may notice reduced lubrication during sexual activity in perimenopause. Some postmenopausal women may not notice changes until several years after their final menstrual period. Once again, the loss of estrogen causes thinning of the vaginal lining, loss of elasticity, vaginal shortening, and diminished lubrication. Vaginal atrophy describes vaginal walls that on examination are thin, pale, and dry and can be inflamed. The results of these changes are pain (dyspareunia), bleeding, and small tears. Women who remain sexually active have less chance of experiencing these discomforts; with regular stimulation, blood continues to flow to the vaginal area. The old adage "use it or lose it" comes to mind in discussions of sexual health and the midlife woman.

Dry eye syndrome experienced by many peri- and postmenopausal women can be another distressing factor in the transition. The most common reasons for dryness are the normal aging process and hormonal changes. Many women find relief from using artificial tears regularly. Another option is closing the opening of the tear drain in the eyelid with special inserts called punctual plugs.

Women frequently complain about the appearance of unwanted hair on the chin, upper lips and breast. Usually this is not a sign of hormonal or nutritional problems, but the higher androgen-to-estrogen ratio in the body. Hair removal techniques include plucking, waxing, electrolysis and laser hair removal.

Women are two to three times more likely than men to suffer from *osteoporosis*. First, a woman's bones generally start out smaller; then, with the drop of estrogen, bone loss begins to accelerate, intestines absorb less calcium, and kidneys excrete more vitamin D. Perimenopausal women need to be identified for osteoporosis risk factors early in their transition. Do family members have osteoporosis or related bone diseases? Sedentary lifestyles, smoking, excessive use of alcohol, low calcium intake, and vitamin D deficiency are a few risk factors to be aware of. Chapter 5 presents a broader view of osteoporosis and treatment strategies.

Cardiovascular disease remains the leading cause of death in women. Before menopause, the odds of a heart attack or stroke are much lower than in a man the same age; after menopause, the gap narrows, and after age 65, as many women as men die of heart attacks. Understanding the risk factors for women and the early warning signals is critical for consumers and health care professionals, as these are very different from those of men. Risk factors are determined by your age, lifestyle, family history, and overall health. The more risk factors, the greater your chances of heart disease. Turn to chapter 5 to determine your risk factors and changes that could lower your risk.

The remaining health risk for women during menopause transition is breast cancer. It is the most common cancer among women, accounting for 31 percent of all cancers in women. It is second only to lung cancer as a cause of cancer deaths, accounting for 15 percent of cancer mortality in women. The lifetime risk of a woman developing breast cancer is one in eight. The good news for women with increased risk is that the chance of surviving five years or longer after a diagnosis of breast cancer is 97 percent.

This chapter has spanned the continuum of body changes for the menopausal woman from hot flashes to breast cancer. The other part of the picture to remember comes from the 1998 NAMS/Gallup Poll of recently postmenopausal women. Respondents said that they felt happier and more fulfilled at this time of their life than at any other. Postmenopause is a time of opportunity, transformation, and growth.

Chapter Four

HORMONE THERAPY

Expect trouble as an inevitable part of life and repeat to yourself, the most comforting words of all; This, too, shall pass.

—Ann Landers

Do you suspect that you may be going through menopause? Take this quiz to assess your symptoms and help you prepare your discussion with your health care provider.

1. Are you over 35?

    a. Yes   b. No

2. Have your menstrual cycles become irregular (lighter flow, heavier flow, or skipped periods)?

    a. Yes   b. No

3. Have hot flashes invaded your life (sudden sensation of heat in your torso and face) or episodes of night sweats unsettled your sleep?

    a. Yes   b. No

4. Has your ability to concentrate or remember things changed?

    a. Yes   b. No

5. Do you have more difficulty falling asleep or feel more tired?

    a. Yes   b. No

6. Has intercourse become painful or vaginal lubrication decreased?

   a. Yes   b. No

7. Have you had an unusual increase of weight, mostly in the abdomen?

   a. Yes   b. No

8. Do you have less desire for or enjoyment in sex?

   a. Yes   b. No

9. Have you had more difficulty with your mood (irritability or sadness)?

   a. Yes   b. No

10. Has your complexion gone through changes (drier than usual, acne, or unwanted facial hair)?

   a. Yes   b. No

A = 10 points, B = 0 points   Total:_____
0–30: You have very few symptoms at this time but stay tuned to your body for the future.
31–70: You do possess some symptoms of menopause; are any causing you stress?
71–100: You have many symptoms of menopause; you may want to share your top concerns with you health care provider.

"A Survival Guide for 'The Hormonal Hurricane'" is provided at the end of this chapter to assist you in those conversations with your health care provider. It is vital that you review your history, research your symptoms, and prepare your questions prior to your appointment. Choosing your provider is the key to your success. Find an individual with an open mind, the right credentials, and good listening skills; then putting the plan into action is up to you.

HISTORY OF HORMONE THERAPY

As some 6,000 women in the United States enter menopause every day, it becomes more of a responsibility for women to be knowledgeable about menopause and to participate with a health care provider in the decision-making process for treatment interventions.

What symptoms are you experiencing?
How disturbing are they to the quality of your life?
What have you tried thus far to minimize the discomfort?
What is your knowledge regarding your treatment options?
What is your preference for treatment?

These five questions should be carefully considered and answered before engaging in a conversation with your provider. Effective communication between patients and providers dealing with clinical decision making has been demonstrated to improve patient care and health outcomes. *Shared decision making* is the new clinical imperative for this century's health care system. To help you be that prepared consumer, this chapter outlines some of the most recent treatment options for peri- and postmenopausal women.

Hormones are a confusing issue for today's consumer, whether they are utilized for contraception, symptom relief, disease prevention, or menopause. Maybe a little jaunt into history can shed some light on the reasons for this confusion. *The Elixir of Youth,* written in the 1960s by Dr. Robert Wilson, a New York gynecologist, began the popularity of estrogen therapy. He was a believer that estrogen might provide the fountain of youth for women. His book ushered in the popular prescribing of estrogen until 1975 when researchers discovered an increase of endometrial cancer and sales hit a low. To counter that trend, physicians prescribed progesterone along with estrogen to help slough the endometrial lining of the uterus and decrease the risk of endometrial cancer. A rebound of popularity occurred with endorsements by celebrities and others as the combined therapy of estrogen and progesterone was thought to lower the risk of heart disease, strengthen bones, and create less chance of developing dementia for women. The 1990s saw annual sales triple. In 1991, the National Institutes of Health began the Women's Health Initiative (WHI) to study estrogen as a preventive medicine for aging women, not just as hormone treatment for menopause. Fourteen million women were on hormone therapy (HT) in 2002 when the estrogen–progestin part of the study was terminated. The study focused on the correlation between HT and risks of breast cancer and other health problems like heart disease. The media reported that women taking Prempro, a pharmacologic combination of estrogen and progestin, were at a higher risk for breast cancer, stroke, blood clots, and heart attack and that they faced a 26 percent increased risk of developing breast cancer. It was an exaggeration of the preliminary reports since the baseline risk of developing cancer in menopause is about 2 percent.[1] Until the end of the WHI in 2002, physicians routinely prescribed HT to protect midlife women against heart disease and for brain and bone health. Other discrepancies or surprises reported in the WHI related to the women selected for the study. The average age of women was age 65 (rather late to begin HT when the average age for menopause is 52), 30 percent of the women in the study were obese, 25 percent were tobacco users, and at the start of the study the participants did not have menopausal symptoms. In August 2003, the Million Women Study from the United Kingdom confirmed the initial WHI study. Since the report in 2002, the number of women using HT has dropped to approximately 6 million and has stayed there. New practice guidelines after the 2002 report recommends that HT be avoided for disease prevention and that its use be limited to menopausal symptom relief in the lowest effective dose for the shortest necessary duration.[2]

Although the media release of the 2002 WHI report seemed to create a panic for women and health care providers either using HT or discussing its potential use, it did stop the general prescribing practice of placing menopausal women on HT routinely. What is the knowledge base of today's woman regarding the risks and benefits of HT? A national online survey in 2004 posed these questions to 781 women. The result claimed that approximately two years after the WHI results were disseminated, women's awareness and knowledge of potential risks of HT were less than satisfactory. The recommendations from this Stanford study suggest that health care providers take the lead in providing education and resources for consumers; that providers stay abreast of the latest research findings about HT as well as alternative nonhormonal, nonpharmaceutical therapies; and that they be prepared to initiate discussions early with women and to a younger, less educated and African American population.[3]

Other important women's studies to focus on hormones and illness are the Nurses' Health Study, the Guttmacher Institute Report, the Postmenopausal Estrogen/Progesterone Interventions (PEPI) trial, and the Heart and Estrogen/Progestin Replacement Study (HERS). In 1976, Dr. Frank Speizer initiated the Nurses' Health Study on the long-term effect of oral contraceptives (OCs). The study, funded by the National Institute of Health, surveyed 59,337 nurses ages 33 to 55 years. Nurses were surveyed every 2 years for 16 years. Investigators found that, among other things, the risk of coronary heart disease was lower in women who chose to use estrogen and progestin. In 1989, Dr. Walter Willet conducted the Nurses' Health Study II (NHS II) to explore the risk factors of major chronic illness in women targeting a younger population ages 25 to 49; they added diet and lifestyle risks. Every year, NHS II prepares an annual newsletter and an archive of the more than100 studies. In 2007, the lead article suggested that memory loss can be delayed by staying physically active, eating vegetables regularly, maintaining a healthy weight, and getting a good night's sleep.[4] The Guttmacher Institute evaluated multiple factors, including genetic and environmental components, that are an influence when menopause begins. Guttmacher's Study of Women's Health Across the Nation of 15,000 women from five racial and ethnic groups recruited women ages 40 to 55. Results demonstrated that women reached menopause sooner if they had a history of heart disease (1.4 years earlier), smoked 10 to 19 cigarettes a day (1.4 years), and reached menopause later if they used OCs and had children.[5] The PEPI trial was a three-year study of 875 healthy women ages 45 to 65 done in 1987 showing a heart-protective benefit of estrogen. The HERS studied 2,763 postmenopausal women with the average age of 67 who had suffered heart attack or chest pain caused by blocked arteries or had undergone heart surgery. Their hypothesis was that estrogen would prevent a second heart attack when, in fact, HT seemed to increase the risk of heart attack and blood clots in the legs and lungs during the first year. A Cochrane review of databases up to November 2004 reviewed the long-term use (at least one year) of estrogen with or without progestins for peri- and postmenopausal women. Their findings concluded that continuous use of HT (combination estrogen and progestin) significantly increases the risk of blood clots, heart attack, stroke, breast cancer, gallbladder disease, and dementia in women. After four to five years of treatment with HT, the study did find a decreased risk of fracture and colorectal cancer. The highest risk of cardiovascular events occurred with combined HT in the first year of use, and HT was not found to be beneficial for routine management of chronic diseases.[6]

From the unfolding of historical perspectives and long-term national studies, various options for women experiencing menopausal symptoms have developed pharmaceutical/medication interventions, herbs or supplements, complementary and alternative interventions, and, most recently, the popular advent of bioidentical HT. Yet history has proven that hormone balance is not a one-size-fits-all proposition. If one goal in this balance proposition is to feel your very best, it makes sense to begin with lifestyle adjustments—changes in diet, exercise, and stress management, to name a few. Then, after lifestyle changes, if you do not have adequate relief of symptoms, short-term interventions beginning with nonprescription supplements are recommended. Although research continues to evaluate the use of supplements for menopausal symptom relief, outcomes are varied; part of the discrepancy may be related to the *placebo effect*. The placebo effect is the positive response a woman may feel from her symptoms based solely on the power of suggestion. The third level of intervention is medication, whether bioidenticals or pharmaceutical prescriptions. The following sections outline each of the categories and provide information for you to discuss with your health care provider.

THE DECISION: SUPPLEMENT, HORMONES, OR WAIT IT OUT

Deciding to take supplements or hormones or to wait it out for symptom relief from the menopause transition can be a daunting process. Many factors come into light at this time: your general health and well-being, your risk factors, the impact of the symptoms on your ability to function, your medical history, your goals for HT, and your general lifestyle. Some women decide to wait out the symptoms since for many they are temporary in nature. Others may try an herbal supplement for hot flashes and for a period of time note some relief. Then the herbal remedy loses its effectiveness as hormone balance becomes more erratic, and a woman may seek professional help and HT.

Hormone testing can be very tricky. One rule of thumb regarding hormone testing is to establish a baseline and provide a guide if hormone treatment is started later on. Blood (serum) testing of hormone levels is only a glimpse of your hormone status at the particular time of the test. Hormones fluctuate from month to month, from day to day, and even from minute to minute since your menstrual cycle and stress level influence what the brain and glands, such as the thyroid, pancreas, and adrenals, will release via hormones into the blood. If blood hormone levels are to be drawn, you have to include where you are in your cycle at the time of the collection. Christiane Northrup, MD, a noted menopause specialist, recommends testing a week before a cycle for perimeno-pausal women, thus obtaining the peak progesterone level and the amount of circulating estrogen and testosterone.[7] Serum or blood testing remains the worldwide gold standard for evaluating women's hormone levels and is rou-tinely used by research groups. Collection should be 7 to 10 days before your next expected cycle or at least 18 days after the first day of your previous pe-riod. Do not take hormones the day of the test. Then resume your hormones following the blood draw. Serum tests should be interpreted in relation to what day of the cycle the blood was collected. Days 1 to 13 of your cycle constitute the follicular phase, and days 14 to 28 make up the luteal phase. Knowing when the blood was drawn and in what part of the cycle you are in will determine what your level should be at that specific time. Try to repeat the levels every three months until balance is achieved, then once annually. Blood levels measure the total amount of hormone, bound and unbound, in the body. Serum consists primarily of water and water-soluble substances like sodium, potassium, and calcium. Sex hormones like estrogen and progester-one are fat soluble, not water soluble; to travel in the bloodstream, they must be bound to a protein molecule. These fat-soluble substances are absorbed from the stomach and gut and then transported to the liver. In the liver, they are attached to a carrier protein that is water soluble and then released into the blood for transport. When attached to a carrier protein, the fat-soluble hor-mones are inactive, or bound. Sex hormone–binding globulin (SHBG) is the major protein responsible for transporting estrogen in the blood. Measuring serum hormones gives you data on how much hormone is in the blood but not on how much is accessible to the tissue or active in the body.

Saliva testing is another reliable test of active, accessible hormones in the body. This method of testing was discovered in 1959 and is widely available; however, it remains controversial for some in the medical community since it is unfamiliar to many physicians. Dr. Northrup is a proponent of saliva testing, as is Dr. John Lee, another menopause expert. They believe that to make a meaningful diagnosis, it is necessary to know how much hormone is available in the body and tissues. Salivary glands possess the unique feature of allowing fat-soluble substances to pass from blood into the saliva in addition to allowing the unbound portion of estrogen to enter into saliva. The portion that is bound to the protein carrier cannot enter. This makes saliva an excellent medium to measure the amount of free hormone available to breast, uterus, brain, and other tissues that are sensitive to sex hormones. The saliva test ordered may require a single vial of saliva or, for a full panel over a 28-day period, multiple vials of saliva that are frozen during the collection. For the woman wanting to determine her ovulation cycle, this 28-day collection is very helpful. (Saliva testing is available through various laboratories; Appendix D offers several suggestions.)

Before beginning any form of HT, a few guidelines are the following:

- Obtain a baseline hormone level
- Determine your goals for treatment but be realistic (you will not be able to prevent wrinkles forever, but you may improve skin's elasticity)
- Begin with the lowest dose for the hormones that need to be balanced
- Annually reevaluate your plan and the need to continue HT
- Optimize your lifestyle: diet, exercise, supplements, and stress management

NONHORMONAL THERAPIES: VITAMINS, HERBS, AND SUPPLEMENTS

The majority of health care providers begin their recommendations to the new perimenopausal woman with encouragement to reevaluate her lifestyle for potential changes that would ultimately ensure a healthy transition. I certainly encourage women to reflect on diet, exercise, management of stress, and identification of a minimum of five coping skills to help them weather the upcoming hormonal storms (for coping skills, see chapter 7). Review the bookshelves at your local bookstore; how often do you see the word "balance" in the menopause section? "Balance your hormones," "balance your life"—it becomes clear that one identifiable action is available for the woman entering "the change": balance. Most women have just spent the past 10 to 20 years living anything but a balanced life, so now you are invited to put on the brakes and coast, not charge forth with new purpose toward balance. This section gives you the opportunity to reflect on your own knowledge, comfort, and readiness to live a life of balance. How balanced is your lifestyle? Do you carve out time to play and refuel your spirit? What percentage of time does your work fill your week? Is a healthy, well-balanced diet the norm for you?

A balanced diet low in saturated fat and high in whole grains, fiber, fruit, and vegetables, with adequate water, vitamins, and minerals, contributes to good health. None of us can dispute this wise recommendation. However, how many women have an ample amount of the necessary vitamins and minerals in their daily diet? Do you know which vitamins and minerals you need for this next phase of life: midlife? Consumers can find the over-the-counter assortment of dietary supplements, vitamins, and natural nonprescription products confusing. In the United States, government regulation of dietary supplements is less strict than that applied to prescription drugs. This lack of standardization opens the consumer to a variation in quality, a potential discrepancy between the amount of the active ingredients listed on the label and the actual amount in the product, and any alteration or contamination of a product. Consumers have been cautioned regarding the strength and quality of products and encouraged to purchase "pharmaceutical grade" or products labeled "USP" (U.S. Pharmacopoeia) or "NSF" (National Sanitation Foundation) in an attempt to limit poor quality control products. The Food and Drug Administration (FDA) established a new rule, effective August 24, 2007, for good manufacturing practices of dietary supplements. The rule will help ensure that products are produced with accurate labeling in a quality manner and do not contain contaminants or impurities. The three-year phase-in allows large and small companies to be compliant by June 2010.

If the human body requires more than 45 vitamins and minerals to maintain health and if daily diets for the majority of Americans arc less than ideal, it stands to reason that a good-quality daily multivitamin with a mineral supplement is a wise action to take. In your younger years, your daily diet probably met most of your vitamin and nutrition needs; however, hormone fluctuation, health conditions, and the normal aging process can hinder the utilization of various vitamins. In those cases where a vitamin or mineral deficiency is noted, the following section can assist in your discussion of options with health care providers.

A brief overview of vitamins and minerals and some of the major food sources where you can obtain them follows:

Vitamin A helps to establish healthy skin, eyesight and immune function.

> Sources: organ meats, sweet potatoes, pumpkin, carrots, spinach, collards, turnip greens, egg yolk, milk, cheese, and butter

Vitamins B1 (thiamin), B2 (riboflavin), B3 (niacin), B6 (pyridoxine), B9 (folate, folic acid), and B12 (cyanocobalamin) assist in the metabolism of amino acids and help fight off heart disease and stroke and possibly improve memory.

> Sources: whole-grain products, meats, fresh vegetables, and fortified cereals

Vitamin C (ascorbic acid) aids in tissue repair, metabolism of hormones, synthesis of proteins, and immune function.

> Sources: citrus fruits, green vegetables (peppers, broccoli, and cabbage) tomatoes, and potatoes

Vitamin D is essential for the efficient absorption of calcium for bone health.

Sources: sunlight exposure, oily fish (salmon), fish liver oil

Vitamin E (α-tocopherol) assists in red blood production and various cell functions.

Sources: nuts, seeds, whole grains, vegetable oil, and wheat germ

Minerals act as biochemical triggers to promote the work of enzymes in the body. The daily requirements of minerals are met for most women with a conventional diet.

Calcium is the most abundant mineral in the human body. It helps to build bones and clear toxins and helps with blood clotting. Calcium decreases with the drop in estrogen production with menopause.

Sources: milk, cheese, yogurt, ice cream, canned fish (salmon and sardines), and green leafy vegetables

Magnesium helps to build bone and increases flexibility.

Sources: nuts, soybeans, cocoa, green leafy vegetables, and bananas

Zinc can be found in almost every cell. It is essential to stimulate the activity of more than 100 enzymes and is needed for DNA synthesis and wound healing, supports the immune system, and helps maintain the senses of taste and smell.

Sources: oysters, red meat, poultry, beans, nuts, whole grains, and dairy products

Clinicians agree that unless a woman has significant medical issues, a premium multivitamin taken daily should meet the majority of a woman's vitamin and mineral needs. The information in this section provides a resource for you to evaluate your current vitamin supplement and your diet regime.

HERBAL SUPPLEMENTS

Some of the more popular supplements for women are soy products, red clover, black cohosh, ginseng, and evening primrose oil. In fact, the debate rages on regarding the benefits of herbal supplements. I do not think providers can dismiss the voices of consumers and the benefits they experience from the use of herbals. Yes, these can have a placebo effect, but, it remains a woman's choice, and an open-minded provider is a definite benefit during this confusing time.

How often have you heard friends swear that soy products help to decrease the frequency and intensity of their hot flashes? The National Institute on Aging is in the process of conducting a major soy study. To date, results are unclear from the scientific world on the true benefits of soy to reduce the vasomotor symptoms of menopause. *Soy* contains plant chemicals called *isoflavones*, which make up one of the three principal groups of *phytoestrogens*, the most studied of the botanicals for menopause-related conditions. Phytoestrogens are plant-based compounds with a chemical structure similar to estrogen. The question remains, How effective are soy protein and soy isoflavones in reducing the multiple concerns for the peri- and postmenopausal woman?

A review of research projects over the past 10 years reveals that there may be some benefit on cardiovascular health because of their inhibiting effect on the progression of atherosclerosis, that a small benefit exists for short-term treatment (12 weeks) of hot flashes, that soy treatment for hot flashes is safe for the breasts and the endometrium (lining of the uterus), but that no strong evidence is reported in the prevention of postmenopause bone loss. Other herbal supplements are the following:

Black cohosh has been used by North American Indians and healers for hundreds of years. European nations have utilized black cohosh to treat menopause-related symptoms for more than 50 years. The marketed brand name is Remifemin, which is used widely in Europe and is a well-documented alternative to HT. The recommended dose is 40 mg/day, with results evident within 8 to 12 weeks.

> *Dong quai,* also known as Chinese angelica, has been used in China for at least 1,200 years. The Chinese use it extensively for gynecologic conditions in conjunction with other herbs, rarely alone. It has been called female ginseng because of its ability to enhance energy and a sense of well-being. Its weak estrogen-like properties has led to its recent resurgence and popularity.
>
> *Evening primrose oil* is promoted to relieve hot flashes, breast pain, and premenstrual syndrome; however, the only research study of 56 symptomatic women with hot flashes found it to be no more effective than placebo in controlling vasomotor symptoms.
>
> *Red clover* (Trifolium pratense) is a rich source of a number of isoflavones, a phytoestrogen that acts like estrogen to relieve menopausal symptoms, to stimulate the immune system, and to treat coughs and respiratory system congestion.
>
> *Flaxseed oil* is another compound receiving media attention for its high concentrations of lignans, phytoestrogen. Data remain mixed as to its effectiveness with menopausal symptoms. Flaxseed is a rich source of omega-3 fatty acids; thus it may have a beneficial effect on cholesterol levels and reduce the risk of heart disease. As with so many of these dietary supplements, further study is warranted.
>
> *Ginkgo biloba* has been used medicinally for thousands of years. Today, it is one of the top-selling herbs in the United States. Ginkgo is used to treat numerous conditions, such as dementia, and for memory enhancement and improving blood flow.
>
> *Ginseng* supplements have been promoted as products for women and men to build stamina and resistance to disease, as aphrodisiacs, as a nourishing stimulant, and to improve thinking and learning. The dosage recommended is 200 mg/day for no more than three weeks at a time, followed by a one- to two-week rest period.

Although women speak highly of the effects of ginseng, evening primrose oil, dong quai, licorice, and Chinese herb mixtures, there are no clinical studies as to their safety, and the North American Menopause Society (NAMS) does not recommend any of them. If you choose to try them, consult your physician, especially if you are on cardiac medications and blood thinners. Why do so many women claim that they work on hot flashes, insomnia, and memory? It could be the placebo effect, thus bringing some relief to an otherwise stressful situation.

BIOIDENTICAL HORMONE REPLACEMENT THERAPY

"New form of hormone therapy sparks debate—Are 'bioidenticals' any safer than traditional hormones?" This was a top news story on NBC Nightly News on November 2, 2006. Dr. Nancy Snyderman, chief medical editor, was interviewing various medical experts and celebrities like Suzanne Somers as to the safety factors for bioidenticals. And for many in the health care industry, it is safe to say that the verdict is still out. Or maybe it depends on whom you talk to. My agenda is to bring you the latest information, both scientific and popular, and to let you take the issue into your own hands and those of your health care provider for "shared decision making."

Bioidentical hormones are chemically synthesized to be identical to the hormones naturally produced in the human body: estradiol, estrone, estriol, progesterone, DHEA (diahydroepiandrosterone), and testosterone. This synthesis is derived from hormone precursors found in soybeans and yams in contrast to the traditional synthetic hormone products given to women over previous decades, such as Premarin, Provera, and Prempro, which are made from animal products developed by pharmaceutical companies. "Bioidentical" and the term "natural" are at times mistakenly used interchangeably when in fact "bioidentical" is the more appropriate term to use to reflect this hormone process. Formulas are prescribed on the basis of the results from the client's saliva hormone testing, the final composition being individualized by the compounding pharmacy.

Bioidentical hormone replacement therapy (BHRT) gained ground in the media after the reports of the WHI in 2002. This study cost the American public more than $628 million and was partially funded by Wyeth-Ayerst, the manufacturers of Premarin and Prempro. Results of the large hormone replacement clinical trial reported cancer- and clot-inducing properties of Premarin and progestins for a percentage of women in the study receiving these drugs. On publication of the WHI results, a large percentage of women stopped HT and went in search of other options for symptom relief. One 2007 study found that 87 percent of the respondents on HT stopped after the WHI report with a concern about an increased risk of cancer or a general increase in risk to health with 26 percent restarting HT, mostly to treat the troubling symptoms.[8] Clinicians believe that BHRT is an option when used short term for relief of menopausal symptoms: hot flashes, mood swings, vaginal dryness, and sleep disruption.

Treatment with bioidentical hormones is based on a unique cocktail of hormones individually designed for a woman reflecting her hormone deficiencies. The major benefit remains the individualized dose prepared in a form to maximize absorption by the body: cream, oral, injections, patches, or suppositories. Although some of the estrogen and progesterone components are

FDA approved, the mixtures are not; they are natural substances prepared by compounding pharmacies. So why are the pharmaceutical companies so distressed by the advent of bioidenticals? Is it all about economics? Bioidenticals are a natural substance; they cannot be patented, and therefore vast sums of money cannot be made from selling the compounds.

Small studies have indicated that these bioidentical hormone compounds are safer than and as effective as synthetic or animal hormones even though they are not FDA approved. It remains necessary to substantiate the findings of these small research studies with long-term, broad population-based research. After the enormous revenue used for WHI, one wonders what hormone manufacturer in the medical or research community would take the financial risk of a long-term study to verify the scientific evidence needed to promote bioidenticals, a nonpatent product? Several well-respected menopause specialists—Dr. Christiane Northrup, Dr. Robert Greene, Dr. John Lee, and Dr. Daniela Paunesky—have endorsed bioidenticals either singly or in combination to maintain the optimal levels of hormones in a woman's body.

Potential advantages of bioidenticals are that individualized compounded doses are prescribed versus a one-dose-fits-all approach, topical administration can avoid some of the problems of orally administered hormones, progesterone may work differently on the surface of the body, and users of esterified estrogen had no increase in venous thrombosis (blood clots). A pilot study conducted by the National Institutes of Health indicated that the risks of blood clotting and strokes that arise from Premarin and PremPro are sharply lowered or nonexistent with bioidentical esterified estrogens.[9]

The downside of bioidenticals must also be presented to enlighten consumers. First, these individually compounded mixtures have not been approved by the FDA; thus, they do not have the rigorous government safeguards that patented drugs must pass. In January 2008, the FDA sent warning letters to seven pharmacy operations that made false or misleading claims about their products. The bottom line from the FDA is that all patients who use compounded HT drugs should discuss menopause HT options with their health care providers to determine their best options."[10] A 2004 NAMS position statement strongly endorses the use of traditional estrogen or estrogen plus progesterone therapy as the best available treatment for menopausal symptoms such as hot flashes, sleep disorders, and night sweats. The NAMS standard of care for menopause HT remains the use of the lowest effective dose for the shortest period of time.[11] A 2005 statement by the American College of Obstetricians and Gynecologists regarding bioidenticals warns that "there is no scientific evidence supporting effectiveness or safety of compounded bioidentical hormone therapy and they should be considered to have the same safety issues as those hormone products that are approved by the FDA and may also have additional risks unique to the compounding process."[12] Finally, a Harvard Medical School health publication acknowledges that studies have shown that bioidentical hormones can help relieve hot flashes and vaginal dryness, but few large studies have investigated the differences among various hormones and methods of administration.[13] More research is needed. Ultimately, Harvard's position is sound: women should work closely with their health care providers to determine what is right for them.

PRESCRIPTION HT

Menopause is as individualized as a thumbprint. Thus, HT should be based on an individual woman's symptoms, which are created by an imbalance of hormones in her body. What time has elapsed since the onset of her menopause? Which symptoms are perplexing her, and what degree of impact do they have on her quality of life? All these issues and her underlying risks need to be explored to rule out concerns with stroke, blood clots, cardiovascular disease, breast cancer, diabetes, bone loss, and other conditions before the onset of HT. Treatment for symptom relief should be at the lowest effective dose for the shortest period of time. In the spirit of shared decision making, a woman and her health care provider work together to determine her goals, risk factors, and the benefits of treatment.

In the pursuit of an optimal hormone treatment plan, women ought to be advised that it takes time to find the best treatment for them, a plan that includes regular reevaluation of hormones and tapering doses. In fact, her HT plan may require more than one product. Peri- and postmenopausal women should be cautioned not to expect immediate relief, as the use of low-dose estrogen or estrogen with progesterone can take 8 to 12 weeks to reach therapeutic levels. Then it is important to initially retest every three months and evaluate the overall plan of care annually. Timing of HT initiation in naturally menopausal women is important. Where is she in the menopause transition? Is this a woman in the late phase of perimenopause experiencing moderate symptoms or a postmenopausal woman in the first five years of menopause? In both cases, HT can be initiated with a low-dose plan. Designers for the WHI study learned that the age of the woman and her place in the transition greatly affect the outcome of HT. They chose older women who did not have symptoms and began HT some 10 years after their assent into menopause. We learned much from their design mistakes. Younger women in menopause— the newly postmenopausal women who begin HT—can find that they are at lower risk of coronary artery disease and that the risk of stroke is lower in women aged 50 to 59 or women starting HT within five years of menopause than for the older woman more distant from menopause. The WHI reports that older women are at a greater risk for heart attack during the first year of HT than are younger women.

Systemic HT, or medications that affect the whole body, remains the most effective treatment for moderate to severe vasomotor symptoms. However, different estrogens, progesterones, and routes of administration (pills, patches, creams, suppositories, and vaginal rings) offer potential advantages for symptom relief when one delivery method or brand of medication does not work fully. An example of this is the perimenopausal woman (her uterus remains intact) with mild to moderate hot flashes, sleep disruption, and irritability; she can begin with a transdermal patch of estrogen and progesterone and avoid the systemic route but still obtain great results. Progesterone is advised for all women with an intact uterus who are using oral estrogen therapy, thereby reducing the risk of uterine cancer.

A decision to discontinue HT warrants a discussion with your health care provider. Although no data definitively support tapering the dose or an abrupt stop, sharing your concerns and taking part in shared decision making makes the health care process more collaborative. Annual monitoring of HT includes an evaluation for potential adverse effects, a review of new research findings, an opportunity to decrease the dose or method of delivery to the most effective one, and a review of other annual testing. Annual mammograms are necessary while on HT.

My intent in this section is not a detailed discussion of all the HT options for women but rather a broad overview of the basic categories, some of the more popular brands and delivery modes, and some of the possible side effects. I hope this will provide a base for your discussions with your provider; if you need further resources, Appendix D provides Web sites and resources to aid you. Estrogen-containing drugs are divided into two categories: estrogen therapy (ET) and combined estrogen–progesterone therapy (EPT). Estrogen therapy, or unopposed estrogen (no progesterone), is often prescribed for the postmenopausal woman who has had a hysterectomy. EPT, a combination of estrogen and progesterone, can be used for the peri- and postmenopausal woman. The estrogen factor offers the greatest benefit for symptom relief; progesterone's job is to oppose estrogen and reduce the risk of endometrial cancer for women with an intact uterus. As an aside, if you are from the old school and remember seeing "hormone replacement therapy" in most of the literature, you will now see "hormone therapy" instead. The FDA declared that the term "replacement" can no longer be used in the marketing of products since the term is a misnomer for this process.

The perimenopausal woman beginning to experience mild to moderate menopausal symptoms may find OCs or birth control pills the first line of HT introduced. These estrogen and progesterone combinations offer not only low-dose hormone replacement but protection from an unintended pregnancy as well. Even though her fertility is in decline, a perimenopausal woman can become pregnant because of the erratic nature of her hormones. These combination contraceptives are safe, effective options for healthy, nonsmoking, midlife women and provide important noncontraceptive benefits: regulation of irregular bleeding, reduced vasomotor symptoms, decreased risk of endometrial cancer, and maintenance of bone density.

Instead of the older traditional OCs that provide 21 active tablets and seven hormone-free tablets, the newer *oral combination contraceptive* options include Lo Estrin-24 Fe or Yaz; these are based on 24 active pills followed by 4 placebo pills. In addition, they cause less breakthrough bleeding or spotting and less weight gain, acne, and mood changes. Before a discussion of extended OCs begins, let me share some terminology: *breakthrough uterine bleeding* is unpredictable and irregular bleeding, while *withdrawal uterine bleeding* is predictable bleeding that often results from progestogen withdrawal.

Seasonale is an extended OC formulation providing relief from monthly cycles but bleeding every three months. Lybel, a newer formula, offers a steady low-dose hormone with no withdrawal bleeding after the first few cycles.

Nonoral combination contraceptives, such as the vaginal ring (Nuva ring) and a weekly patch (Ortho Evra or Evra), are worn for three or four weeks and result in cyclical monthly withdrawal bleeding.

Progestin-only contraceptives offer an option for perimenopausal woman who smoke, who are over the age of 35, who have hypertension, and who have a history of venous thromboembolism, or blood clots, in the leg. They are available as oral tablets, injections, subdermal implants, and intrauterine devices. The downside of this type of OC is that women may experience irregular bleeding, spotting, or *amenorrhea* (absence of menses). Injectable progestin-only contraceptive provide an effective, long-term contraception when the hormone is delivered in a suspended solution (depot). Depo-Provera is an injection given every three months; the newest form, Depo-subQ Provera, contains less progestin and is injected subcutaneously into the thigh or abdomen every three months using a smaller needle, causing less pain. Initially, some irregular bleeding may be experienced; after four or more injections, at least one-half of women will experience amenorrhea.[14] For a woman in perimenopause with irregular cycles, there are few vasomotor symptoms, yet wanting freedom from monthly periods, this is a reasonable option—an option your mother never had.

Implanon is a toothpick-sized subdermal implant of progestin only that is placed under the skin of the inner arm and offers highly effective contraception and hormones for up to three years. Norplant, another implant offering up to five years of contraception, is no longer available in the United States.

Intrauterine devices offer highly effective, long-term, and convenient contraception. Mirena is a popular option for women with a five-year period of contraception. Unfortunately, the irregular bleeding and spotting reported by women creates a downside for some. The copper intrauterine device (Para-Gard T 380A) is approved for 10 years of contraception. The side effects are increased cramping and menstrual flow.

Cautions noted for perimenopausal women who are considering estrogen-containing contraceptives are the following:

- Current or past coronary artery disease
- Cerebrovascular incidents
- Valvular heart disease
- Diabetes mellitus with vascular concerns
- Uncontrolled hypertension
- History of breast cancer
- Active liver disease
- Cancer of the endometrium
- Thrombophlebitis
- Headaches with auras
- Undiagnosed abnormal genital bleeding
- Obesity
- Cigarette smoking
- Prolonged immobilization

Samantha is a 54-year-old woman who began experiencing mild hot flashes five years earlier and was placed on OCs. Her vasomotor symptoms have been relieved. Recently, she has experienced gastric distress, bloating, and reflux symptoms. She is concerned that the OCs may be causing her problems. Samantha decided to stop her OCs, and her hot flashes, night sweats, and sleep disruption returned. After testing her hormones, she decided with her health care provider to try a continuous combination transdermal patch (low-dose estrogen and progesterone). How is the decision made to transition from using hormonal contraception to lower-level menopause HT? At age 55, approximately 90 percent of women will have reached menopause. Many clinicians use this target age to transition women from OCs to HT. A woman's risk–benefit analysis is an initial step in the transition process. The cautions cited previously are reviewed along with family history; the menopause phase and symptom intensity to determine the preferred HT. Another component to consider is a woman's need for the short-term relief of symptoms or long-term therapy for the prevention of disease.

Estrogen therapy takes into consideration the type of estrogen (human, nonhuman, synthetic, and plant based) the severity of symptoms (mild, moderate, or severe), medical factors (vaginal atrophy, osteoporosis, and liver function), delivery method (oral, transdermal, cream, vaginal rings, or suppositories), and a woman's individual needs and preference. In chapter 2, three types of human estrogen occurring naturally in the body were discussed in detail: estrone, estradiol, and estriol. The *nonhuman estrogens* refer to conjugated estrogens, a mixture of at least 10 estrogens obtained from natural sources (the urine of pregnant mares) that occur as sodium salts of water-soluble estrogen sulfates. *Synthetic estrogens* are produced as esterified estrogens and synthetic conjugated estrogens. Another recent estrogen option on the market consists of designer estrogens known as *SERMS* (selective estrogen receptor modulators), which bind with estrogen receptors and selectively modulate the effects of estrogen in different body tissues. Tamoxifen is the oldest; it blocks the estrogen receptors on breast cells while maintaining some positive effects on bone, uterine tissue, and the cardiovascular system. There are not enough long-term studies to assess their benefits and risks, so you may want to avoid using SERMS or limit their use until more evidence is made public.

Exploring the pathway that estrogen takes from swallowing a pill to the point that estrogen benefits the body is worth a short discussion. Estrogen is well absorbed in the gastrointestinal tract after taken orally and is metabolized in both the gut and the liver before reaching the general circulation in the body. This is called the *first-pass effect*. This pathway does decrease the amount of estrogen available for circulation. By contrast, nonoral routes do not have the first-pass affect through the liver; transdermal and topical preparations cause less variability in blood levels and require smaller total doses than oral therapy, a significant issue for those with high cholesterol and triglyceride blood levels.

The most widely used conjugated estrogen for clinical studies and HT is Premarin. It has been on the market for more than 65 years and is available in oral tablet, vaginal creams, and injectable formulas. Premphase and Prempro have combined progestin with estrogen. Although for years the standard dose was 0.625 mg/day, recent studies confirm a benefit at a lower dose of 0.45 or 0.3 mg/day.

Estradiol is the most widely used estrogen in Europe and the one estrogen available commercially in government-approved formulations that can be considered bioidentical.[15] Estradiol is available as an oral product (Estrace), a transdermal reservoir patch (Estraderm), a matrix patch (Alora, Climara, Estradot, Vivelle, and Vivelle-Dot), a transdermal spray (Evamist), and a topical emulsion (Estrasorb) and in vaginal forms (Estrace Vaginal Cream, Estring Vaginal Ring, Femring, and the vaginal tablet Vagifem).

Transdermal and topical administrations of estrogen have several advantages. Estrogen can be delivered at lower doses than oral administration and are not subject to first-pass liver metabolism. Transdermal administration does not increase triglycerides and has less adverse effect on gallbladder disease and coagulation factors. When estrogen levels need to be monitored, transdermal and topical administrations provide a more stable serum/blood level. One disadvantage of a patch is the adhesive, which can create skin irritation for some women. *Vaginal administration* of estrogen provides for the use of creams, rings, and tablets. Creams are helpful when a small amount of estrogen is needed to treat vaginal atrophy or vaginitis.

Estrogen Functions in the Body
- Regrowth of the uterine lining
- Maintain vaginal and bladder tissue health
- Decrease bone loss
- Stimulate breast cells
- Responsible for fat storage
- Sustain mood, cognition, and concentration

Progestogen therapy in menopause is done primarily to oppose estrogen in women with an intact uterus, thus reducing the increased risk of endometrial disease and cancer. The term "progestogen" refers to a broad range of hormones that resemble natural progesterone in the body, both progesterone and synthetic *progestins*. Progesterone is produced by the ovaries after ovulation and by the placenta during pregnancy. Progesterone that is compounded identically to the body's progesterone is bioidentical, whereas progestins are synthetic and have a progesterone-like activity but are not identical to the body's progesterone. Some progestins are derived from plants (wild yams and soybeans), but because they go through a chemical reaction during synthesis, it is inappropriate to classify them as natural. Provera is the best-known progestogen to deliver endometrial protection; in combination (conjugated estrogen + progestogen), Prempro and Premphase are used. Transdermal progestogens have the metabolic advantage of avoiding first-pass liver effects. Prometrium is an oral capsule containing micronized progesterone suspended in peanut oil; however, caution is raised with women allergic to peanut oil. Compounding pharmacies make micronized progesterone available in creams, lotions, gels, oral capsules, and suppositories. Mirena provides an intrauterine delivery of progestin.

Estrogen–progesterone therapy is classified into several regimens: cyclic, cyclic combined, continuous cyclic, continuous long cycle, continuous combined, and intermittent combined. This can be confusing terminology, but in essence this language refers to estrogen and progestogen compounds in the product (first word = estrogen, second word = progestogen). Cyclic EPT is the oldest method. Estrogen is taken from day 1 to day 25 of the calendar month with progestogen added the last 10 to 14 days. The normal menstrual cycle is mimicked to include ovulation, thus protecting the endometrium. A drawback is that about 80 percent of women have withdrawal bleeding, and some experience vasomotor symptoms. Continuous-combined EPT was designed to address withdrawal bleeding, which is problematic for women and can decrease compliance with HT. This method provides estrogen and progesterone every day, and some women after several months of HT experience absence of menses. The overall goal of EPT is to protect the endometrium, maintain the benefits of estrogen, and minimize uterine bleeding.

Several side effects are possible with estrogen therapy/EPT (strategies are listed):

- Fluid retention (restrict salt, maintain water intake, and exercise)
- Breast tenderness (caution with chocolate and caffeine, lower estrogen, switch estrogen, and switch to another progestin)
- Nausea (take meds with meals or before bed, switch to another oral estrogen, switch to nonoral estrogen, and lower estrogen or progestogen)
- Headaches (restrict salt, caffeine, and alcohol; switch to nonoral estrogen; lower estrogen/progestogen; and ensure water intake)
- Bloating (switch to low-dose nonoral estrogen, lower progestogen, and switch to another progestin)
- Mood changes (rule out depression or anxiety, ensure water intake, lower progestogen, switch progestogen, and restrict salt, caffeine, and alcohol)

Testosterone therapy for women remains controversial. Testosterone is known as an androgen. Androgens are the immediate precursors for estrogen biosynthesis. Even more important are the effects that androgens have on sexual desire, muscle mass and strength, distribution of adipose (fat) tissue, energy, and psychological well-being. Testosterone and DHEA are the two androgens discussed in this section. Both are produced in the ovary and adrenal glands; other sources are the skin, muscle cells, and brain. Women begin with about 20 times less the amount of testosterone than a man; then, between the ages of 20 and 45, a woman's level drops by about 50 percent. Studies show that the decline results from the decreased production by adrenal glands and ovaries, from the general aging process, or from adrenal insufficiency (adrenal burnout). Natural menopause does not have a significant effect on testosterone; however, surgical menopause with removal of the ovaries reduces testosterone by 50 percent. Potential benefits of androgen therapy are improved sexual interest, sensations, and satisfaction. There are no FDA-approved androgen-containing prescription products to treat sexual disorders in women. Research is attempting to remedy this problem, and off-label options are increasing for women. Estratest has been available for more than 40 years but is not officially FDA approved for androgen therapy. Androderm and Testoderm (both in patch form) and Androgel are available for men, but they are not supported by the FDA for use with women. Compounded testosterone products are available for women, although there are not sufficient studies to determine effectiveness and safety, making many clinicians hesitant to prescribe these compounds. One intervention to improve libido is compounded topical 2 percent testosterone USP cream or ointment applied directly to the vagina and clitoral area or on the inner thigh several times a week. Testosterone is well absorbed through the skin. Unfortunately, no controlled studies support this therapy for safety and efficacy, although many anecdotal reports support the use. A recent Cochrane review examined the benefits and risks of adding testosterone to HT for peri- and postmenopausal women. Although the impact of adding testosterone for perimenopausal women remains unclear, there appears to be improvement in sexual functioning in postmenopausal women and is associated with a reduction in HDL (high-density lipoprotein) cholesterol.[16] Several testosterone patches, gels, and other androgen products are under review to improve sexual satisfaction for postmenopausal women. It remains a matter of time and of how much support these products receive in the process.

DHEA remains available as a dietary supplement and can be purchased without a prescription. It is a precursor of testosterone, meaning that the body converts this hormone secreted by the adrenal glands (90%) and ovaries (10%) into testosterone. At age 25, DHEA has peaked in a woman, levels slowly decline after age 30, and by 70 years of age it is almost undetectable. Menopause creates another decline in DHEA production. The studies available evaluate the use of DHEA to treat adrenal insufficiency; other reports indicate an increase of physical and psychological well-being, energy, immune function, and libido with DHEA use. A recommendation of oral DHEA at 25 to 50 mg/day is well tolerated by older women.[17] Some clinicians prescribe topical DHEA 5 mg/ml/day to enhance sexual arousal. DHEA therapy is a new horizon for women's health, and time and research initiatives will tell the story. A rich discussion of DHEA and sexual health can be found in chapter 8.

ANTIDEPRESSANTS AND RELIEF OF MENOPAUSAL SYMPTOMS

Women who have been on HT over several months and still suffer symptoms of hot flashes may want to consider adding antidepressants, such as selective serotonin reuptake inhibitors (SSRIs) and serotonin-norepinephrine reuptake inhibitors (SNRIs). In addition, women who have breast cancer and cannot take hormones may find relief from hot flashes with SSRIs. Effexor (ventlafaxine), Paxil (paroxetine), and Prozac (fluoxetine) provide relief from hot flashes, and women can feel a difference within two weeks. However, the side effects include sexual dysfunction (retards orgasmic function) and sleepiness and may interfere with other medications. Caution is advised for women taking tamoxifen who want to consider SSRIs or SNRIs. Paxil can cause weight gain and may be difficult to discontinue without withdrawal symptoms. Discontinuation of SSRIs should be with tapering, not abruptly, or withdrawal symptoms can occur. Gabapentin (Neurontin) is an anticonvulsant drug that can also assist in treating hot flashes. Initial treatment at a daily dose of 300 mg/day is advisable. Bedtime is the best time to take this drug, as dizziness and drowsiness are possible. If hot flashes do not subside, an increase to 300 mg twice a day or up to 300 mg three times a day may bring results. Antacids may reduce the effectiveness of Neurontin, but do not take the medication for at least two hours after an antacid. Neurontin can cause weight gain, and tapering for discontinuation is always advised. Clonidine, an antihypertensive drug known as Catapres, may be used for mild hot flashes. It is not as effective as the SSRIs and can lower blood pressure, heart rate, and pulse rate and have adverse reactions of dry mouth, drowsiness, constipation, and sedation. Initial dosage is 0.05 mg twice a day and requires a tapering for discontinuation.

A plethora of options for perimenopausal and menopausal symptoms exist. Regardless of the treatment selected, the plan should be periodically evaluated to determine if it remains necessary, as vasomotor symptoms are temporary and new research is evolving frequently.

A SURVIVAL GUIDE FOR "THE HORMONAL HURRICANE"

Now you are ready. What questions perplex you regarding your hormonal health? Have those hormonal hurricanes left you screaming with frustration, kept you up most of the night, and left you wondering what alien life force has taken over your body? This is your opportunity to find the best health care provider for your personality and hormonal needs. It is vital you review your history, research your symptoms, and prepare your questions prior to your appointment. Choosing your provider is the key to your success. Find an individual with an open mind, the right credentials, and good listening skills; then putting the plan into action is up to you.

Begin Your Data Gathering with the Following

- Your medical history: allergies, surgeries, pregnancy history, daily medications, and dietary supplements
- Medical records: take them with you to your first appointment
- What medical conditions do you have? (hypertension, elevated cholesterol levels, diabetes, asthma, depression, or anxiety disorders)
- Has stress been a significant issue in your life? What do you do to cope with stress?
- Do you have a family history of heart disease, breast cancer, osteoporosis, or cancer?
- Did you have significant premenstrual symptoms? How did you deal with them?
- How long have you been perimenopausal? (irregular menstrual periods, hot flashes, night sweats, sleep disruption, or change in sexual desire or lubrication)
- What have you done to deal with your perimenopausal symptoms?

- If postmenopausal, how did you deal with your transition, and what were your concerns?
- Do you have some specific treatment methods you want to discuss?

Now identify the "Top Two Concerns" you have for your hormonal transition. Trying to address more than two issues in the initial meeting is a mistake.

Evaluate the Chemistry with the Provider

- Did the health care provider listen attentively?
- Were questions answered?
- Did you feel rushed or comfortable with the overall session?
- Did you leave with some recommendations or "next steps"?
- Did you make a follow-up appointment?

Chapter Five

REINVENT THE PHYSICAL YOU

You don't get to choose how you're going to die, or when. You can only decide how you're going to live. Now!

—Joan Baez

The "now" part of this chapter's quote is your call to action. Could this be any better a time in your life to evaluate your health potential? Did you notice that I did not speak of the medical problems you may be facing or the changes to your body from the shift in hormones? This call to action is in the spirit of your health and the possibilities that await you—now—an opportunity to gather the forces of what you have learned along the way and how you have lived and to maximize your sense of purpose for the decades that follow. That may mean weeding out habits, styles of living, and even people to promote your new quest to live life fully.

Dr. Henry Lodge, an internist, gerontologist, and author, notes that after the mid-fifties, 70 percent of aging is controlled by lifestyle—sleep patterns, physical activity, diet, and the use of alcohol and tobacco—how you live your life. His seven rules of fitness suggest exercising six days a week, watching what you eat, and caring and being committed to living well. His scientific findings establish exercise as the master signaler that triggers cells to repair and strengthen muscles and joints. Exercise produces other positive actions: changes in brain chemistry, improvement of the immune system, and resistance to diseases such as heart attack, stroke, hypertension, and even Alzheimer's disease.[1] Dr. Lodge recommends at least 20 minutes of aerobic exercise a day to counteract the body's natural decay process and to increase the metabolism, inducing the chemical reactions needed to stimulate new cell growth.

Another reliable source encouraging healthy lifestyles is the U.S. Prevention Services, which declare the improved control of behavioral risk factors, such as the use of tobacco, alcohol, and other drugs. Exercise and nutrition can prevent half of all premature deaths, one-third of all cases of acute disability, and nearly all cases of chronic disability.[2] Imagine the positive benefits of increased productivity and a decreased economic strain on society as mature adults foster healthy behaviors. This could be another legacy of the current generation of seasoned women entering menopause. Women have been known as the "carriers of culture," but I am imagining this generation setting the stage for a culture of healthy, vibrant women who do more than survive through menopause—they thrive.

LIFESTYLES: PHYSICAL ACTIVITY

Begin your *lifestyle assessment* reflecting on physical activity, nutrition, substance use, stress management expertise, and risk factors. Regular physical activity beyond preventing aging disorders can assist in maintaining mental well-being and physical strength. Approximately one-third of American women age 45 and older participate in no leisure-based physical activity. Regular participation in physical activities for at least 30 minutes five or more times a week is recommended, yet fewer than 20 percent of menopause-aged women invest in this lifesaving mode. There are three basic types of exercise:

- *Strength training* includes resistance exercises using resistance bands, free weights, or weight machines. Older women benefit from this type of exercise, as it slows bone loss, builds strength, and improves balance.
- *Aerobic exercise,* such as jogging, brisk walking, cycling, and biking, boosts the metabolism, thus burning more calories and supporting a healthy cardiovascular and respiratory system. Midlife women utilizing low-impact aerobics or elliptical machines place less stress on their joints.
- *Flexibility exercises,* such as Pilates, yoga, tai chi, and stretching, keep the body limber, reduce stiffness, and improve overall flexibility and balance, which may help reduce falls and fractures.

Determine what your current level of activity is, the status of your physical condition, and your exercise preferences before just jumping into an exercise program. It is always advisable to consult your provider before beginning a new regime to prevent injury. Then begin slowly with the aim of 10 minutes a day or 10 minutes several times a day and build your endurance to a minimum of 60 minutes three times a week or, for weight loss, six times a week. The key to your success is the regularity of the workouts. Research shows that it takes up to eight weeks to establish a new habit. I encourage my clients to adopt regular physical activity into their routines for the rest of their lives to ensure a healthy future.

Tips for Success

- Increase your physical activity daily by taking the stairs, parking your car farther from a building, and walking.
- Commit to a gradual but consistent exercise plan,—maybe 10 minutes of walking—and build it by 10 minutes every three to five days.
- Put your exercise plan on your weekly schedule and make it as important as a doctor's appointment.
- Join a gym and commit to three to five days a week.
- Hire a personal trainer for six months to help you keep your commitment.
- Keep your gym bag in the car or a set of workout clothes at the office.
- Talk a friend into being your "workout partner" for support.
- Keep DVDs at home with Pilates, yoga, dancing, and other forms of exercise.
- Vary your workout so you do not get bored; it also helps the body not get bored.
- Keep a workout journal that includes beginning weight, body fat measurements, and training plan.
- Have fun—listen to your iPod and books on tape or do the treadmill while you are watching television—but commit to activity for the remainder of you life.

NUTRITION

There is no substitute for a *healthy diet*. Midlife women have grown up in the era of fast foods and in the land of diet delights: South Beach, Atkins, Beverly Hills, Cambridge, Grapefruit, Jenny Craig, LA Weight Loss, Low Carb, Nutrisystem, Pritkin, Scarsdale, Zone, and Weight Watchers. Can you even open a magazine or read the paper without the testimonials of dieters? How many of these diet trends have you attempted? Where did you have success?

As you assess this part of your lifestyle, you might choose a more sustained approach for your dietary needs, creating a new relationship with food. I still believe that the best mantra for today's midlife woman is "Eat to live, not live to eat." Your nutritional needs can be met through a diet high in whole grains, fiber, vegetables, and fruits and low in saturated fats and cholesterol. As for dietary supplements, they just cannot replace healthy eating. Choosing food you like to eat and not feeling deprived is an important part of your successful, new relationship with food. This requires portion control and the use of moderation. That means you don't have to totally give up your comfort foods; just change the eating habit to a few bites instead of an entire bag of chips or cookies. Vegetables and fruits are a better snack option than that piece of candy, soft drinks, or chips and dip. In fact, it has been shown that any kind of vegetable slows cognitive decline even more than fruits. Eating two or more servings a day decreases the decline in mental processing by 35 percent over six years.[3] So the veggies and dip I keep at the office for a quick snack between clients is a good plan.

Consuming fish, especially oily fish, at least two times a week is another good strategy for healthy eating. The omega-3 fatty acids in fish clean your arterial system, reduce triglycerides in the blood, and decrease blood pressure. Best choices are eight ounces of salmon, mahi-mahi, catfish, flounder, tilapia, and whitefish. Limiting your intake of saturated fats and cholesterol and replacing meat-based meals with vegetable alternatives or fish increases your heart-happy living. Dietary specialists also encourage a minimal intake of beverages and foods with added sugar and caffeine. Caffeine-containing drinks (coffee, tea, and colas and other soft drinks) can trigger hot flashes, contribute to insomnia, and increase dehydration in the peri- and postmenopausal woman. In addition, reducing salt intake can prevent hypertension or facilitate better control of your blood pressure. General dietary guidelines for women and older adults are as follows: 1,600 total calories/day; carbohydrates: 45 to 65 percent/day; protein 10 to 35 percent/day; fiber 25 to 30 g/day; cholesterol 300 mg/day; and sodium no more than 2,400 mg/day.

Alcohol consumption should be in moderation according to the American Heart Association, which recommends limiting consumption to two drinks a day for men and 1 drink a day for women. I had to research this discrepancy on women's behalf. Apparently, when alcohol enters a woman's bloodstream, it reaches a higher level than a man's who may be drinking the same amount. The alcohol is less diluted in a woman's body because she has less total water than a man's. So the rule of thumb is that a "drink" equals 12 ounces of beer, five ounces of wine, or 1.5 ounces of spirits. This little less known fact, regarding the difference between men and women, increases the importance of another thing one must do for healthy living: drink those eight glasses of water a day to sustain your hydration.

The base of the food pyramid for most women growing up in the 1950s and beyond seems to have been fast-food consumption, which has led to increased weight gain, insulin resistance, diabetes, hypertension, and heart disease. Women add an average of one pound a year during perimenopause. Thus, strategies to manage weight for the peri- and postmenopausal woman are essential. The best advice is to eat less and exercise more. Eating a healthy diet while balancing the amount of food you take in with the amount of physical activity you use to burn the calories consumed becomes a wise general rule.

One reason it becomes easier to gain weight and more difficult to lose weight is the fact that metabolism slows at midlife. The fat distribution seems to have found new homes in your belly, hips, neck, and back—a distressing issue for many women and a profit base for the plastic surgeons. On the bright side, recent studies show that eating dark chocolate may lower blood pressure and increase HDL (high-density lipoprotein) cholesterol (the good cholesterol) and lower LDL (low-density lipoprotein) cholesterol (the bad). That little stash of dark chocolate you hide for those special moments you no longer have to hide.

These days you cannot discuss midlife weight control and health risk without understanding the body mass index (BMI), which is the ratio of your height to your weight. Three categories divide the BMI chart: healthy weight (BMI of 19–24), overweight (BMI of 25–29), and obese (BMI of 30–40). Generally, overweight means that you are at least 10 percent above the ideal weight for a woman of your height and weight. But BMI is only part of the story; another gauge at midlife is your waist size, which measures your abdominal fat. More than 35 inches increases your risk of health problems (40 inches for a man).

STRESS MANAGEMENT

Midlife women face many changes—hormone irregularity, the onset of medical conditions, and relationship pressures—all of which can provoke high levels of *stress* affecting your quality of life. How you handled stress in previous stages of life is one indicator of your manageability. You may require a more diverse set of skills now to balance the mind, body, and behavioral challenges. A 2002 study reported more than 52 percent of American adults use mind–body interventions for stress reduction.[4] Mind–body therapies include prayer, coping skills, relaxation, cognitive-behavioral therapies, imagery, and hypnosis. Chapter 7 presents a multitude of options; your effectiveness in diffusing stress will be based on your insight into the early detection of stress and applying techniques to minimize the grip of stress.

RISK FACTORS AND DISEASE

A woman's risk factors during menopause transition are dependant on several components: genetics, hormonal fluctuations, lifestyle, and general aging. Heart disease is the number one killer of women, although most believe that cancer makes the big hit. Heart disease affects women as much as men, and the symptoms are very different but all the more dangerous because they are underestimated.

Cardiovascular Disease

One in three women has some form of cardiovascular disease (CVD). According to the American Heart Association, heart disease and stroke kill approximately 480,000 women every year, and worldwide CVD causes 8.6 million deaths every year. A surprising fact for many is that CVD kills nearly 12 times more women than breast cancer with the rate in women rising slightly over the past two decades, while CVD has declined steadily in men. Heart disease should be on the international women's health agenda, but it is not. Thus, the education of consumers and health care providers becomes everyone's responsibility. A recent survey found that fewer than one in five physicians knew that more women than men die from heart disease and stroke every year. Most clinicians assume that women experience the same symptoms as men before and during a heart attack: crushing chest pain and pressure, tingling down the left arm, shortness of breath, profuse sweating, and light-headedness.[5]

Not being aware of the differences between risks and symptoms creates a major barrier to prevention, diagnosis, and treatment. Women have vague complaints and milder symptoms, and often their electrocardiograms are nonspecific. The most frequent warning symptoms of an acute myocardial infarction are unusual fatigue, sleep disturbances, shortness of breath, weakness, indigestion, and anxiety, which may be present for more than a month before a myocardial infarction. These symptoms are often misdiagnosed as indigestion, gallbladder disease, depression, or anxiety.

Fortunately, heart disease can be prevented with better nutrition, fitness programs, smoking cessation, improved drug therapy for hypertension and high cholesterol, and an informed public. First, educating the public to the major risk factors for CVD—obesity, high cholesterol, hypertension, diabetes mellitus, smoking, sedentary lifestyle, and family history—is a step in the right direction. Second, it is important to provide information on preventive measures to forestall the disease process of CVD. Finally, women need to be educated regarding the differences in their symptoms and the need for early intervention. Women of color are particularly at risk of CVD as diabetes; hypertension and high cholesterol are more prevalent.

And what of the debate regarding hormone therapy (HT) and women's cardiovascular health? Is it harmful? The 2002 report of the Woman's Health Initiative ended early because participants were found to be at greater risk for coronary heart disease. After reinvestigation and closer scrutiny of the participants selected, HT does not seem to increase CVD risk in women unless they had established CVD to begin with. Other results showed a lower cardiovascular risk in women who begin HT near menopause or five years after the final menstrual period. It is still too early to advocate HT for CVD prevention for all women; studies are under way. In the meantime, decisions about HT should be made on an individual basis, weighing the risks and benefits for the individual woman and, if started, beginning with a lowest dose possible for a limited period of time. A successful education program to assist in delivering the message of healthier hearts is Heart Truth for Women of the National Heart, Lung and Blood Institute. The number of women struck by heart attack can only decline with an educated health care system and consumers who are aware of their risk factors and symptoms.

Metabolic Syndrome

Metabolic syndrome has become increasingly common in the United States, affecting approximately 25 percent of the population. It is known in other medical circles as syndrome X or insulin resistance syndrome. The syndrome is a cluster of conditions that occur together, increasing your risks of heart disease, diabetes, and stroke. Having just one of these conditions does not give you the diagnosis, but it does contribute to your risk for the disease. The metabolic risk factors include abdominal obesity (excess fat tissue in and around the abdomen), high triglycerides, low HDL, high LDL, elevated blood pressure, and insulin resistance.[6] Insulin resistance is a disorder in which the body can't use insulin efficiently. Other conditions increasing your chances of metabolic disorder are physical inactivity, aging, hormonal imbalance, and genetic predisposition.

Once again, lifestyle therapies are the first-line interventions to reduce the metabolic risk factors. They include weight loss to achieve a BMI less than 25, increased physical activity with a goal of at least 30 minutes of moderate-intensity activity on most days of the week, and healthy eating habits that include reduced intake of saturated fat and cholesterol. Diagnosing women with this syndrome is critical to help identify aggressive lifestyle modifications and focus on weight reduction and medication if necessary. We do know that a woman with a high BMI (between 18.5 and 24.9 and waist circumference of more than 35 inches) is prone to more frequent and intense hot flashes; thus, diagnosis and treatment are important to improve her quality of life.

Diabetes Mellitus

Type 1 diabetes mellitus (DM) is often called "insulin-dependent" diabetes. It is usually diagnosed in children and young adults. It occurs when the body does not produce enough insulin, a hormone needed to convert glucose (sugar), starches, and other food into energy needed for daily life. Type 2 DM is more likely to develop in men and women as they age and is called "non–insulin-dependent" DM or "adult-onset" DM. Although type 2 DM remains undiagnosed in approximately one-third of women, 12.5 percent of women aged 50 to 59 have DM, and the rate increases to 17 percent at age 60. Another unsettling point is that women with type 2 DM are at higher risk for developing CVD, which also increases with age. Complications of uncontrolled type 2 DM include loss of vision, kidney failure, neuropathy (nerve damage), and amputation. Thus, screening for diabetes is important and in fact is recommended for all women over age 45. Glucose screening with a fasting plasma glucose test is done at a medical facility. However, type 2 DM is often not diagnosed until complications appear. Studies do show that menopause does not lead to increases in impaired fasting glucose.

An intensive lifestyle modification program has been shown to delay and sometimes prevent the onset of type 2 DM. For women at high risk, decreasing weight, combined with at least 150 minutes of exercise a week, can decrease the risk by 58 percent.[7] Other interventions for the diabetic woman are management of glycemic control (glucose levels), lipid control (HDL and LDL), blood pressure, and HT. Women with type 1 or 2 DM present a clinical challenge when hormones are needed for either contraception or menopause therapy. Women with menopausal symptoms seeking relief would benefit from transdermal therapy, as it does not increase triglyceride levels and seems to have less effect on gallbladder disease and blood clotting in the venous system. If estrogen and progesterone therapy is needed for the woman with type 1 DM, it is suggested that exposure to progestogens be minimal. The important point is that if you have a risk factor for DM, the best avenue consists of lifestyle modifications.

Osteoporosis

The old saying "an ounce of prevention is worth a pound of cure" should be a menopausal woman's theme song for prevention of *osteoporosis*. Currently available treatments only halt bone loss; they do not rebuild bone. Building up your reserves of bone before you start to lose it during perimenopause sets you up to weather the storm of bone loss and to prevent a trip to a rehab center after hip fracture. Osteoporosis is often called the "silent disease" because bone loss occurs without symptoms. Women may not know they have osteoporosis until their bones become so weak that a sudden strain, bump, or fall causes a fracture. Fractures of the vertebrae, bones of the spine, and the hip are the most common and lead to a national health care cost of approximately $10 million per year to treat. Your bones are made of living, growing tissue with two continuous processes: the breakdown and the formation of new bone tissue. A person normally builds more bone than he or she loses until about age 30. During the aging process, bone begins to break down at a faster pace than it builds up, and the loss of estrogen in perimenopause hastens brittle bones even further. Risk factors include age (there is a decline after age 30) gender (a woman over age 50 is four times more likely to develop osteoporosis than a man), being white or Asian (these populations are more at risk than women of color), and being petite and thin women. A family history of osteoporosis increases your risk as well.

You can slow bone loss with adequate intake of dietary calcium and vitamin D, exposure to sunlight, and physical exercise. A postmenopausal woman needs up to 1,500 mg/day of calcium. Excellent sources are milk and dairy products, salmon, dark green leafy vegetables, and foods fortified with calcium. Supplements are generally needed only if you do not get enough calcium in your diet, so consult your provider. Your body uses vitamin D to absorb calcium. Being out in the sun some 20 minutes a day helps the body make the vitamin D it needs. You also get vitamin D in eggs, salmon, cereal, and milk. Another must to decrease the impact of aging on the bones is a regular exercise program, along with weight-bearing exercises, done at least three to four times a week, such as walking, jogging, playing tennis, or dancing.

Preventive steps include limiting alcohol consumption and not smoking. Some medications, such as steroids, anticonvulsants for seizures, blood thinners, and thyroid drugs, can lead to more bone loss. To determine if your bones are weakening, a painless and accurate test can provide you with valuable information. The bone mineral density test is an X-ray used to determine bone measurements. It is usually indicated for women age 65 or older, women with numerous risks, or menopausal women who have had fractures.

Treatment involves HT and a variety of medications established for osteoporosis. Hormone therapy is believed to be useful for postmenopausal women in preventing or alleviating the increased rate of bone loss. Estrogen saves more bone tissue than even large daily does of calcium, but it is not without risks for other problems like breast cancer, gallbladder disease, blood clots, stroke, and heart disease. Women unable to take HT now have another option: bisphosphonates and calcitonin. Bisphosphonates are a group of medicines used to prevent or treat osteoporosis; they slow bone loss, increase bone density, and reduce the risk of spinal fractures. Actonel, Fosamax, Boniva, and Didrocal are a few examples; they are considered the first line in treatment. Most women have seen the commercials by known celebrities supporting the once-a-month dose of Boniva for bone loss. Since adherence to osteoporosis therapy is so poor, a once-a-month oral tablet has increased compliance with women. Calcimar, a naturally occurring hormone involved in calcium regulation, also helps to slow bone loss. It is marketed as Miaclcin, a nasal spray used daily. Evista (raloxifene) is a selective estrogen receptor modulator (SERM), meaning that it has many of the properties of estrogen and is known to target specific problems, in this case bone loss.[8] Finally, if you have osteoporosis, you need to protect yourself against accidental falls. Making your home safe means keeping it clutter free and removing loose items and rugs; installing grab bars on tubs, showers, and by the toilet; and installing proper lighting.

CANCERS

After heart disease, cancer is the second-leading cause of death for women. Nearly 80 percent of all cancers are diagnosed at age 55 and older. Women have a one-in-three lifetime risk of developing cancer.[9] Although menopause is not responsible for an increased cancer risk, the aging element of menopause becomes the culprit. As part of an annual physical exam, it is important for women in menopause or over age 55 to be evaluated for risk of cancer of the breast, lung, uterus, ovary, colon, rectum, and skin.

Tobacco use, alcohol use, poor nutrition, and lack of exercise are behaviors that increase your risk for cancer. In the United States, 85 percent of lung cancer is due to smoking. Smoking is also related to risk for cancer of the mouth, throat, and cervix. About one-third of all U.S. cancer deaths are attributed to diet and obesity.

Breast Cancer

Breast cancer has the highest incidence for women, with the single most important risk factor being age. A woman's lifetime risk is one in eight and increasing with age. About 70 percent of women diagnosed with breast cancer each year are over age 50, and almost half are age 65 and older. Other risk factors include an immediate family member with breast cancer, having cancer in one breast, late menopause (after age 55), starting menstruation early (before age 12), having a first child after age 30, or never having children. Although the incidence of breast cancer has increased in recent years, the mortality rates have decreased. It is hoped that this is due to early detection from the use of mammograms, self-breast exams, and maybe medical research having identified several potential cancer-causing genes, including BRCA1 (linked to breast and ovarian cancer) and BRCA2 (associated with breast cancer and postmenopausal ovarian cancer). During self-breast exams, warning signs are any change in the nipple or breast, lumps, any change in the contour or rippling of breast skin, any discharge (clear or bloody from the nipple), and persistent redness or scaliness or a retracted nipple.

Some recent studies report a greater increase in breast cancer with combined estrogen–progesterone therapy (EPT) than estrogen therapy alone. The North American Menopause Society's 2007 position statement on HT is that breast cancer risk is increased with use of EPT beyond five years.[10] We do know that most women initiate HT for relief of vasomotor symptoms that are often temporary; thus, it is important once relief is obtained to taper off as soon as possible. Women with breast cancer are vulnerable when it comes to debilitating menopause-related symptoms and relief. Alternatives to HT should always be tried first, and the decision must be made with a woman's full awareness that therapy may promote more rapid tumor growth. Tamoxifen was the first SERM noted in 1960 to prevent initiation and promotion of breast cancer; it did, however, stimulate the growth of endometrial cancer.

The Food and Drug Administration's black box warning was advised in 2002 for uterine malignancies, stroke, and pulmonary embolism. Raloxifene, another SERM used for osteoporosis, has been found to significantly reduce the incidence of postmenopausal breast cancer. Research has made leaps in the past 20 years for breast cancer, but we still have a way to go.

Endometrial Cancer (Uterine Cancer)

Uterine cancer affects the cells that line the outside of the uterus-endometrium. It is the fourth most common cancer for women after breast, lung, and colon cancer. It is usually detected early because it produces vaginal bleeding between menstrual cycles. If discovered early, this slow-growing cancer is usually confined to the uterus and can be surgically removed often eliminating all the cancer. Your first clue that something is wrong is abnormal vaginal bleeding or any bleeding after menopause or pink, watery discharge. A Pap test does not detect this cancer. To sample cells of the endometrium, a biopsy from inside the uterus is taken, or a transvaginal ultrasound (wand inside the vagina) may be used to detect other conditions. Once found, a staging is done to determine surgical treatment and involvement of other areas. Surgery is the most common treatment with an aggressive form; additional treatments may be necessary, including radiation, HT, or chemotherapy. Having strong supports during diagnosis and treatment is paramount.

Cervical Cancer

The mortality rate of cervical cancer has dropped sharply over the years because of the Pap test. Studies show that virtually all cervical cancers are related to infection by sexually transmitted infections, human papillomavirus (HPV) being the most recent infection in U.S. women age 15 to 59. Cancer that forms in tissues of the cervix (the organ connecting the uterus and the vagina) is usually a slow-growing cancer that may not have symptoms but can be found on a Pap test. Pap tests take tissue by scraping the cervix and looking under a microscope for abnormal cell growth. Risk factors include infection with HPV, early sexual contact, multiple sex partners, cigarette smoking, and oral contraceptives when women take them longer than five years. Cervical cancer usually does not cause pain; the most common sign is abnormal vaginal bleeding or discharge. Diagnosis requires a cervical biopsy; colposcopy, or examination with a microscope to inspect the cervix for abnormal cells after staining with a harmless dye; the LEEP technique, which uses an electrified loop of wire for a tissue sample; or cone biopsy, which removes a cone-shaped section of the cervix. Precancerous cells may be removed via procedures such as LEEP, cone, and, when required, hysterectomy, the most invasive treatment.

Most women diagnosed with precancerous changes are usually in their twenties and thirties. For the earliest stage of cervical cancer, more than 90 percent of women survive at least five years after diagnosis. Early detection remains the most effective approach to cancer of the cervix.

Ovarian Cancer

Ovarian cancer is a malignant tumor within a woman's ovaries and causes more deaths than any other cancer of the reproductive system because it is usually detected in an advanced stage. The first sign is usually an enlarged ovary. Other symptoms include swollen abdomen, low abdominal pain, change in bowel habits, bloating, fatigue, urinary tract symptoms, or pelvic pain. These symptoms often confuse a woman who may already experience bloating or abdominal pain from gas, distention, or gastric distress. The involvement of the urinary system is a differentiating element to alert a woman that the symptoms are more than stomach distress. Studies show women who have children and breast-fed or who used oral contraceptives are less likely to develop ovarian cancer.

Colon Cancer

Colon cancer is cancer of the large intestine (colon). Approximately 112,000 people are diagnosed annually by colonoscopy. Most cases begin with a small, noncancerous polyp without symptoms. Signs of colon cancer are often change in bowel habits (diarrhea or constipation), blood in the stool, persistent cramping, gas or abdominal pain, weakness or fatigue, and unexplained weight loss. Risk factors are long-standing inflammation of the colon (such as ulcerative colitis), Crohn's disease, genetic syndromes, diet low in fiber, sedentary lifestyle, diabetes, obesity, smoking, heavy use of alcohol, and age (90 percent are older than 50). Screening begins with fecal occult blood (an annual test to rule out blood in the stool), digital exam, sigmoidoscopy (use of a flexible scope to examine the rectum and lower colon), and colonoscopy (a flexible fiber-optic device to see the large intestine and allow for removal of polyps). After age 50 and with average risk factors, a colonoscopy should be done every five years and more frequently when polyps are found. Survival is directly related to detection and the type of cancer involved.

RECOMMENDED HEALTH SCREENING
FOR THE SEASONED WOMAN

If this chapter has led to one awakening, let it be the vital importance of lifestyle and decreasing risk for disease or, on a positive note, your key to vibrancy for the following decades. What subtle changes can you make? Are there modifications that can increase your health status or nullify some risk factors? Remember that it takes a good eight weeks for a new activity to become a habit. And you do not have to begin all out: what about those 10 minute walks, building by 10 minutes every three to five days? One study even suggests more benefit in three 10-minute exercise appointments than one 30-minute activity.

Annual Screening to Sustain Your Health

Complete physical exam	Pap test with pelvic exam	Breast exam
Cholesterol	Skin test: moles	Blood sugar
Fecal occult blood	Mammography (after age 50)	Dental exam and cleaning
Eye exam (test for glaucoma)		

Baseline Studies to Help for the Long Term

Bone mineral density	Electrocardiogram
Sex Hormone panel	

Chapter Six

REINVENT THE EMOTIONAL YOU

It's never too late to be what you might have been.

—George Eliot

A patient recently shared a story of discovery with me. She was sitting in the reception area, awaiting her monthly hair-coloring appointment. As usual, the area was rich with magazines; *People, Glamour, House Beautiful,* and *Health.* But one particular article caught her eye; the headline read, "Menopause— Beginning Your Next Three Decades with the Right Spirit." The article mentioned the fact that American women reaching 54 years of age can expect to reach 84.3 years of age. So a good one-third of life is lived after reaching menopause. Her realization was that she indeed had much living to do. Ann had recently celebrated her fifty-eighth birthday about the same time her youngest daughter moved out of the house. She and her husband of four years had a welcomed period of adjustment, only to discover that they enjoyed the quiet of less "girl drama," fewer phone calls coming into the house, and the ability to pass by the daughter's vacated room and see the floor.

So now what? Many questions ran through her mind—it seemed like simultaneously. How *am* I doing? How do I feel about reaching this phase in life's journey? What would I have done differently? What am I glad I have done? What do I want to be sure I do not miss in the next part of the journey? If I could enter a new career, what would it be? What kind of mother-in-law and grandmother will I be?

At the next week's therapy session, I invited her to slow down a little. Her daughter is only 19 and not even dating a special man, and her son is just finishing college and very single. Let's start with, How do you feel about reaching this point in your journey, before you enter grandmotherhood? In therapy, she was exploring her low sexual desire as a by-product of perimenopause and becoming more comfortable with the body of a 58-year-old woman. So the magazine article only helped distill the need to examine "reinventing the emotional self" for her.

You too may have seen articles like the one mentioned previously that catch your breath or books on the bookstore shelf that you must pick up and scan, all with the purpose of making you rethink where you are in life, who you are, and what you want to do with those marvelous years remaining. I am reminded of a fabulous book I picked up at the bookstore some two years ago: *Sex and the Seasoned Woman: Pursuing the Passionate Life,* written by Gail Sheehy. I was intrigued by the title. Her groundbreaking work with *Passages* and *The Silent Passage* were on my bookshelf; what new discoveries has she made? Leaving the bookstore with my parcel neatly wrapped, I waited to get home to discover the midlife revolution for the boomer-generation women she writes of. No one says it better than Sheehy: "A seasoned woman is spicy. She has been marinated in life experiences. Like a complex wine, she can be alternately sweet, tart, sparkling, and mellow. She is both maternal and playful. Assured, alluring, and resourceful. She is less likely to have an agenda than a younger woman—no biological clock ticktocking beside her lover's bed, no campaign to lead him to the altar, no rescue fantasies. The seasoned woman knows who she is. She could be any one of us, as long as she is committed to living fully and passionately in the second half of her life, despite failures and false starts."[1] How many women had crossed my office threshold with the desire to be fully connected to their physical, emotional, and sexual self? I could relate to the premise of Sheehy's book, and I had to agree that the second adulthood is indeed more freeing than the first. So the challenge resides within each woman to tap into that seasoned woman and reinvent all three domains of life—physical, emotional, and sexual. This chapter focuses on the emotional wealth that awaits you.

THE EMOTIONAL YOU

The emotional you is an outgrowth of all the opportunities, relationships, challenges, failures, and successes encountered along the way to becoming you. This chapter provides techniques to unearth a view of the past, models to examine options for the future, and strategies to support future endeavors for your ongoing success and fulfillment. This will not be a therapy session, but it will be more of an open dialogue with yourself.

In the recovery community, people in "the program" are often cautioned not to "take another's inventory." However, for our purposes, this is your opportunity to *take your own inventory*. Your inventory or story includes the various life cycles—the challenges faced, difficulties encountered, and successes accomplished. The My Story Exercise in Table 6.1 lists the various life cycles: infant, toddler, school-age child, adolescent, young adult, mature adult, and seasoned adult. For each cycle, there are potential peaks and valleys—stories you heard about the family, your behaviors, challenges you faced, difficulties you encountered, and the successes gained.

Directions given to my clients are to find some alone time when you will not be interrupted. Carve out at the most 30 minutes to an hour and begin the visit with *you*. Use the My Story Exercise to provoke memories and information. Enter each life cycle with curiosity and history as a companion. For example, under "Infant," you can address what your family told you of your arrival. Were you planned? Did Mom have any difficulties with the pregnancy or delivery? Did your infant years progress with normal developmental milestones: walking, talking, cutting those first teeth, and so on? You might write, "I was planned and loved and grew up as the second daughter."

Adolescence can provoke more details, stumbling blocks, and even traumas. Several of the women I work with hit a wall in adolescence regarding their sexual development; a few even experienced a "sexual stall-out." Patty came to work with me at age 39. She loved her husband of 17 years, Pat. But she could no longer wrestle the uneasiness that came when he made sexual overtures. When she was five years old, her father had touched her inappropriately; when she told Mom, she was told, "That could not be." Years progressed, and she found Dad looking at her with a weird look. "It made my skin crawl," she said. As a teenager, he would come into the bathroom when she was in the tub or just enter her bedroom without a knock. Doors were locked, and she kept her silent vigil. Mom turned a deaf ear to her concerns, so the conversations stopped. A "developmental stall-out" occurred, interrupting her sexual

Table 6.1
My Story Exercise

Life Cycles	Challenges	Successes
Infant		
Toddler		
School-age child		
Adolescent		
Adult		
Seasoned adult		

development. Early in her relationship with Pat, she knew she could tell him her story and be heard. He heard Patty but expected her to be a willing and warm sexual companion: "After all, you have been in therapy. You said the demons of sexual abuse were banished. Why can't you just have fun and be sexual with me? I'm your husband, not your father."

Patty wanted to move beyond the uneasiness of being sexual with Pat. Even though sexual abuse work with a therapist can release the demons for some clients, sex therapy may be needed to move beyond the stall-out. Patty discovered her "sexual self" in our work. Then she and Pat learned how they could blaze new trails for sexual connection. Patty's stall-out came to light when she began her work and used the My Story Exercise. I remember her telling me at the onset of our work that I was her third therapist and that she had worked for years with a clinician who helped her deal with the abuse from her mother's denial and her father's betrayal but still felt uneasy being sexual. The My Story Exercise gave her the opportunity to discover the stall-out and grieve her lost sexual self.

This exercise is a quick inventory, not a novel to be written. Some joys can come to light, while disappointment may also sneak up on you. Should painful memories remain, talk with someone supportive to process them or find a therapist for some focused work.

DETERMINING NEEDS AND WANTS

Another exercise that can unlock emotional barriers on the path to reinventing the emotional you is the Needs and Wants Exercise in Table 6.2. Many people have difficulty differentiating a *need* from a *want*. And I must admit that in my young adult years, I thought they were synonymous. In the 1980s, when I was doing a good deal of recovery work with individuals in my practice, I discovered Pia Melody's work and soon learned the difference between the two. Those were the years when clients wanted to heal from codependency, dysfunctional families, and addictions and champion their inner child. I continue to find the exercises from that era beneficial with clients. People often come in for therapy at midlife wanting to know who they are, what they need and want now, and how to make the necessary shifts to obtain that well-being. The Needs and Wants Exercise is a classic in my therapy repertoire (see Table 6.2 and 6.3 for this valuable exercise). I use it on an annual basis to give my own life direction.

Let's begin with some definitions. *Needs* are those things you must have to survive, a bottom line, a necessity for the safety and security for an individual. Legitimate dependency needs for adults are food, shelter, clothing, medical and dental attention, physical nurturing, emotional nurturing (time, attention,

Table 6.2
Needs and Wants Exercise

Need (to survive, must have)	Big Want (moves life to well-being)	Little Want (preferences, brings joy)
•		
•		
•		
•		
•		
•		

Table 6.3
Life Factors to Consider Related to Your Needs and Wants

Family	Social	Physical
Intellectual	Emotional	Growth
Safety/security	Career/job	Spiritual
Relationships: friends, etc.	Leisure	Sexual

and direction), sex, and financial security, which includes earning, saving, spending, budgeting, and investment needs. Pia Melody further distinguishes *wants* as "big wants" and "little wants." A big want takes your life in a general direction of well-being and brings fulfillment, while little wants are things we do not have to have but are preferences or bring joy.[2]

Some issues for individuals that make it difficult to acknowledge and meet needs and wants are the following:

- *Being too dependent*—They know what needs and wants are but expect others to take care of them or wait in expectation that their needs will be met.
- *Being antidependent*—They can acknowledge needs, try to meet them, find that they are unable to ask for help, or would rather go without what is needed or wanted than to be vulnerable.
- *Being needless and wantless*—They have needs and wants, but they are not aware of them.
- *Needs and wants get confused*—They know what they want and get it, but they do not know what they need.

The Needs and Wants Exercise is great for couples who are planning a marriage or are stuck in a power struggle. The exercise helps them see clearly when they are on the same track as a couple or need further discussion to understand the other's perspective and desires. I recently shared the exercise with John, a widowed man who was building a new life with Lisa, a woman who was also widowed. They had been lifelong friends and found love with each other later in life. The exercise gave them a concrete forum in which to discuss their individual lives and the future.

I began by explaining the exercise, gave them a handout with the definitions, and used the flip chart to draw three columns ("Need," "Big Want," and "Little Want") and then subdivided each of the three categories with their names. They took turns sharing either a need or a want while I charted it on the paper. A list of life factors from the handout gives specific components of life that each can relate to (see Table 6.3). For example, the physical, intellectual, emotional, social, family, and spiritual factors have an impact on life. A "need" for Lisa was to see her family at least twice a year. A "big want" she acknowledged was the desire to travel once a year for vacation. Did she "have to have" a vacation, No. But the excitement of planning the excursion with her partner and exploring new places together created more intimacy and well-being for the relationship. Once John heard and understood this, he could get on board and stop complaining about the money that would be spent. And a "little want" that brought Lisa joy was going to movies at least once a month. The specific and measurable nature of the exercise helped John learn more about her and their compatibility. One murky area was his "need" to save money each month, while Lisa knew very little about saving. An outcome from the exercise was that John and Lisa visited their financial planner together and drew up a plan based on needs and holdings. What could have been a rift was diverted by an exercise and an action plan.

ENGAGING YOUR SECOND ADULTHOOD

Okay, seasoned woman, you have some exercises to address where you have been. And you have explored one model to assess needs and wants. Let me make a pitch for you to regard Sheehy's notion of the second adulthood and her research in the five phases in pursuit of passionate life. First adulthood began when you left the security of your parent's home to become accountable for your decisions, relationships, work ethic, and ultimate well-being. Sheehy states that first adulthood is from ages 30 to 50. She describes first adulthood as follows: "We survive by figuring out how to please and perform for the powerful people who protect and reward us: parents, teachers, mates, and bosses. But by our mid-forties, we are all looking for greater mastery over our environment-emotional, physical, and vocational. It is in her fifties that a woman is fully ready to speak with her own voice."[3] The ushering in of second adulthood provides this vocal, insightful woman an opportunity to scan the environment with new eyes dwelling on the future and being optimistic and purposeful in pursuit of "the passionate life." That is exciting. The potential to reinvent the self, anticipate options, and execute a plan can make "breaking through glass ceilings" look like child's play for these boomer divas.

Initially, I thought that Sheehy's range for first adulthood, ages 30 to 50, was rather old, that a few women may indeed mature earlier than this. Then again, when she wrote *Passages* in the mid-1970s, society had not encountered the baby-boomer generation and their ability to reshape every life cycle they enter. "Midlife" for women then could begin in the mid-thirties. Ask boomers today, some 30 years later, "What is old?" and they tell you "old is 80 plus." More than 60 million boomer women, the earliest of the generation, celebrated their sixtieth birthdays in 2006. And their cry, loud and strong, is, "Sixty is the new 40!" Second adulthood is a time of managing the environment you live in—an environment that includes family, friends, bosses, partners, career, financial responsibilities, leisure opportunities, and homemaking activities, to name a few.

What dreams, ambitions, and passions await you in these years of "transition and vitality"? Are there leisure activities, artistic venues, and creative roles you considered in those early years but did not have the time, energy, or finances for that you would love to pursue now? Now is not too late. The boomer woman entering menopause is just beginning her second adulthood, and with that strong voice, support from friends, and role models who have gone before her, this exhilarating period is a reawakening.

Sheehy's research began with a simple questionnaire on her Web site with the headline, "Sex for Women over 50 Is for the Birds, Right?" You must read her book *Sex and the Seasoned Woman* and meet the wonderful women who revitalized their marriages and found new love, sex, intimacy, dreams, and spirituality as they pursued the passionate life. She found some women who were bold and perceptive who began preparing for second adulthood in their forties. Sadly, she discovered, more women won't think about the reawakening of their life until they are catapulted into upheaval via menopause, medical conditions, children leaving home, the loss of a close friend, or the loss of a loved one through divorce or even death.[4] My hope is that you won't wait but will be proactive and tap into those dreams or passions now.

Let me share a brief summary of Sheehy's five phases in the pursuit of the passionate life. I won't do it justice, so pick up the book and read for yourself. My intention is to have you say, "I can relate to that phase. How do I make it happen for me?"

Phase I: The Romantic Renaissance, or Pits to Peak) (Ages 45–49)

This phase is marked by something or someone sending an "electrical charge" into your world. If you are paying attention, whatever the source, you will be reminded of the powerful woman you are and find an outlet for this "renewed energy." The outlet could be a new vision for yourself, a new vocation, a new dream, a new relationship, a new focused pastime, or a new spiritual focus. The good news is that you have embarked on the passionate life. The bad news is that the "romantic passion" is often short lived, so pay attention and act.

Phase II: Learning to Be Alone with Your New Self (Feisty 50)

"Once the initial passion of the romantic rush wanes, and before you can embrace your full power as a seasoned woman, you will need to spend time alone," Sheehy warns. For the majority of women who have been surrounded by people they are responsible for, this phase may cause a shudder. Be of good faith. Take this as legitimate time to reexamine everything in your life—who you are and who you want to be remembered as. This is a time to shed out-grown roles and responsibilities and abandon the "shoulds." When was the last time you took *you* out to dinner or on a trip or pleasured yourself sexually? Sheehy found that her respondents' success in this phase was noted by "an understanding that you can take care of yourself." Let this second phase widen your imagination for your future and the possibilities that await you.

Phase III: The Boldness to Dream (Selective Sixties)

Carl Sandburg states, "Nothing happens unless first a dream." What is your dream? Possibly, it is a passion from early days to draw, play an instrument, volunteer for a group you hold special in your heart, or maybe travel and live in a motor home. You may be fortunate to share your dream within a marriage and have it validated. You could find a friend or group of people who can ignite your passion. My challenge to you is to embrace it and make it happen.

Phase IV: Soul Seeking (Spontaneous Seventies)

With the shadow of mortality as a backdrop, many enter this phase ac-knowledging a dramatic change in needs and perspectives.[5] Restless souls look for a spiritual connection, some desire a "giving back" to the next generation, and others become more prayerful during this phase. It is a different kind of "love relationship" that is desired now, a deeper soul connection with someone who respects the "pilgrim soul" coined by Yeats. It could be a mate who ap-preciates the "changing face and body," a true friend, or a potential partner, or some may even rekindle an old flame. In my years as a therapist, I have met a number of people coming together in their seventies to share those later years. Some want to revisit their sexual needs that lay dormant because of an aging partner's inability to be sexual, and with the loss of that partner, those dormant desires rise again and have an opportunity to find a loved one to share them with. These are brave souls wanting to share life.

Phase V: Graduating to Grand Love (Enduring Eighties and Noble Nineties)

If the second adulthood dream is integrated into your new life, then your confidence and self-control are abundant. Relationships flourish with a partner, adult children, grandchildren, and those you choose to share time with. Grandparenthood allows you to revisit the wonder of childhood days. A broader view of life and a shorter time to live provide the impetus to give creatively or philosophically or to realign one's goals.

I enjoyed Sheehy's portrayal of the "seasoned siren"—she can enchant both older and younger men with her stories, vitality, wit, sass, and sex can be enlivened by the fact of having more free time.[6]

Let me share the story of Ginger. Ginger was indeed a seasoned siren at the age of 89. Ginger also happened to be my mother-in-law and a remarkable woman who lived that role up to her last days. Professionally, her nursing career had sparked controversy when at age 65 she was to retire from the emergency department. Physicians and staff began a petition in that Canadian province to change the law and not force retirement at age 65—that law should have been called the "Ginger declaration," for she worked another 5 years. On retirement, she headed the Alzheimer's Society, an association she had great passion for after George, her husband, died from this illness. While championing this cause, she met her second husband and even outlived him. I fondly remember one of our last conversations. Ginger told me, "Women are fine. I just prefer the company of men. Oh and by the way, have you found me a nice man for the next time I come for a visit?"

I can honestly say that various women have been significant role models for me during my life, and I am grateful for them all. Ginger will always the premiere model of the "seasoned siren." My desire for each of you is that you gracefully or passionately embrace these phases with renewed commitment to live your life fully.

MONITORING MOODS

In the first two sections of this chapter, I shared techniques to unearth the view of the past or your story. Then two models to examine options for the future were presented: the Needs and Wants Exercise and Sheehy's five phases in pursuit of the passionate life. The following section highlights strategies to help you make the future an ongoing success. Strategies such as mood evaluation, coping skills, leisure skill building, relaxation, meditation, spirituality, and friendships can greatly enhance the future for the seasoned woman.

Mood and emotion are often used interchangeably, yet are they the same? I think not. Emotions are those fleeting or temporary feelings that arise from an event, a thought, or even a person. Catch a brilliant sunset over the lake, feel the emotion of joy or peace, and maybe even excitement. Hug your daughter who has been gone from you for some time because of angry words. What emotions come forth: relief, gratitude, or surrender from the hurt? Moods seem to run deeper in the psyche. They can have a positive or a negative effect on your feelings and even your sense of well-being. You might have awakened on the wrong side of the bed. Describe the mood and the impact on your day—that impact can last a few minutes or a few hours or for some all day long. Just ask a parent of a teenager enmeshed in a relationship drama. One day not so long ago, I felt like walking on eggshells in my own home as my then 17-year-old daughter struggled with the "Shniggins," the name given to the group of girls she hung out with in high school. Dramas often flamed through our home like wildfire: "Who said what to whom?" "Who ignored who in the lunchroom or talked to the wrong person about the wrong thing on the phone?" My ongoing fantasy was that all their cell phones would lose their signal for a whole week without the daily drama.

Hormones and mood are strange bedfellows. The body's hormones are connected to one another just like the spheres on a beautiful mobile that hangs from the ceiling on your porch—each hormone and its system represented by the color cylinders are linked to one another via the golden thread. Watch a gentle breeze come through the room and what happens to this balanced mobile: it shifts a little. Notice the movement of the mobile as a strong wind blows through the room: it spins and dips, each cylinder in flux. Your mood also shifts a little during the course of a week as the environment you live in and your hormones interact with each other. Perimenopause and menopause are more like the "strong wind" blowing through the room—hormones are more in flux because of the highs and lows of the sex hormones, so the mood state also fluctuates. When estrogen levels are low, a depressive mood can ensue. Yet high levels of estrogen with a sagging progesterone level can add to an anxious state, while the elusive testosterone of perimenopause, when elevated, provokes irritability. Without a balance of the sex hormones, mood and emotion can stimulate behaviors that may seem extreme for the situation. Once again after work, your partner goes next door to visit with the neighbor's husband before coming home to say, "Honey, I'm home!" You stick your head out of the sliding door and yell, "So are you coming in *this* house, or do you plan on spending the few hours we have together with the damn neighbor?" How many times have you felt surprised by your own behavior when the situation did not appear that upsetting just moments before?

As a psychiatric clinician, individuals with *mood disorders* pepper my appointment book. Mood disorders are prolonged moods that affect the individual's life at work at home, socially, and with activities of daily living such as eating, sleeping, and moving about. Anxiety and depression are mood disorders that are dramatically affected by sex hormones. Think back to early adolescence, premenstrual episodes, and postpartum periods: the sex hormones are irregular during these times of hormonal flux, often leaving a woman feeling depressed, anxious, or totally unlike herself. A portion of the emotional unrest is derived from environmental influences, such as the upheaval of an adolescent's desire for freedom or the arrival of a new baby into the family, yet the hormonal hurricane is evident for the woman and the people who interact with her.

Midlife, another major turning point, can usher in many life issues that some are ill prepared for: launching children into the world, an elderly parent's care-taking needs, body changes with aging, medical concerns, the end of fertility, career factors, and relationship demands of partners, friends, and family or possibly divorce and even widowhood. Because moods can change in response to the fluctuating hormone levels of estrogen and progesterone, a woman in the menopausal transition is at risk for mood disorders. If you have attempted to negotiate the rough waters of depression earlier in life but fell prey to a mood disorder, another risk factor is added: stress. However, I believe that the way one *perceives* stressful issues and the *variety of coping skills* on hand to mediate stress are the two biggest equalizers of stress (discussed later in this chapter). Mood, hormone fluctuations, genetics, past bouts with depression or anxiety, stress, and environmental and relationship challenges add up to a major challenge for the resilience of the midlife woman.

Stress is inevitable in today's fast-paced and often demanding world. How do you perceive stress? Is there a cumulative pattern of stress in your life? What have you done to weather the storms of stress in the past? What strategies were successful, and which were not? In my own life, a major stress currently in operation is the deadline for this manuscript to the publisher's office. Oh, and did I mention that it is the week before Thanksgiving and the beginning of the holiday season? So what is my perception of this stress, the environmental impact, strategies that worked in the past, all are factors that can set me up for success, failure or a bout of depression or perhaps anxiety? My perception is that stress is not an uncommon force in my life, nor has it been debilitating for me in the past. I have a wealth of coping skills at my fingertips that have helped me weather the storms of stress (my favorites are music, daily affirmations, journaling, and exercise). The environmental impact—the holidays—is here; it will happen, and I cannot put it off, but I can ask for help and include family members in the planning and execution of the celebration. Again, perception is important: I enjoy the holidays and do not want this season remembered as "2007 holiday horrors and the manuscript." So I will tailor my expectations for myself and the season, the outcome being enjoying family and friends, while at the heart of my success is self-discipline and an action plan.

Effective educators generally take a pretest of participant's level of knowledge or skill set at the onset of an educational endeavor and then enroll participants in a posttest preceding the educative experience. Your mood pretest is given in Table 6.4. For the next month, you can monitor your *mood state* and the *adaptation* you employ to determine whether there is a mood disorder, whether your stress level is creeping up on you, how much your hormone depository or cycle affects your mood, and whether your coping skills are effective in modulating the impact. Every other day, chart whether your mood has been affected by the symptoms listed on the exercise, the coping skill you utilized, and the benefit achieved.

By the end of the month, your mood and adaptability will be very clear. If there is a need to seek professional help from a health care provider, you have concrete information to share. At the very least, you will know what coping skills you possess and their effectiveness or a warning signal to broaden your skill base. Take heart: chapter 7 provides a plethora of copings skills to help you weather those hormonal hurricanes.

Table 6.4
Mood Adaptability Cycle

Symptoms	Mood (R, S, O)	Coping Skill (identify)	Level of Benefit (1–5)
1. Irritability			
2. Fatigue			
3. Forgetfulness			
4. Insomnia			
5. Angry outbursts			
6. Depression			
7. Anxiety			
8. Crying spells			

Over the next month, every other day, chart if your mood has been affected by the symptoms listed here, the coping skills utilized, and the benefit achieved.

Mood impact: (R) rarely, (S) sometimes, (O) often
Coping skills: exercise, relaxation, music, talking to someone supportive, prayer or negative copers such as eating, sleeping, drinking to excess, yelling, pouting
Level of benefit: from coping skills, 1–5 rating (1 = low benefit, 5 = high)

DEPRESSION

Depression, those feelings of sadness, hopelessness, and despair, are not a predictable outcome of menopause. However, having a solid understanding of depression, one's predisposition to depression, the types of depression, and potential treatment options can take away some of the mystery and fear regarding this mood disorder.

From the exercise identified earlier, you may find that your well-being is solid or possibly hampered by multiple days of irritability, sadness, and hopelessness. Let me start the discussion of depression by sharing some known facts. Many women in perimenopause from ages 45 to 55 describe this period as some of the best years of life. Recall the statistics from earlier chapters: 20 percent of women have no significant change other than a gradual cessation of menses, 50 percent display mild discomfort from symptoms, and 30 percent have considerable discomfort that affects the quality of life. So let's focus for a moment on those 50 percent of women with moderate effects. They may find themselves sad at times and bothered by some but not all symptoms or maybe bothered by symptoms but for short intervals. Women whose emotional makeup is sensitive to hormone changes are often more symptomatic or even clinically depressed. As a clinician assessing the vulnerability of women in menopause for depression, I refer to their history for level of risk. A woman with one previous episode of diagnosed depression has a 50 percent chance of a second depression. Those who have experienced two episodes of depression are at a 70 percent risk of depression reoccurring, and a woman is 90 percent at risk if she has been depressed three times in her life. Hot flashes are a second factor predisposing women to depression. Perimenopausal women who have experienced hot flashes are four times more likely to become depressed than those who have not. A study conducted by Massachusetts General Hospital in Boston[7] revealed that estrogen is the common denominator in the equation of reoccurring depression and hot flashes. Estrogen levels during perimenopause wax and wane, producing unstable levels of serotonin, a neurotransmitter needed by the brain to assist in mood regulation.

It is important to understand estrogen balance and its relationship to neurotransmitters in the brain. Estrogen can assist the brain in signaling and regulating messages to other parts of the body. But it is the *serotonin,* one of the best-known neurotransmitters, that helps regulate mood, sleep, depression, and anxiety. Other neurotransmitters are dopamine, norepinephrine, and acetylcholine. It is the balance of the neurotransmitters, the brain's messenger system from neuron to neuron, that helps to level mood state.

As a psychiatric nurse practitioner, I have seen how a little bit of serotonin can improve premenstrual symptoms and relieve women from wanting to pull out their hair, yell at the kids, and rant at her husband. There seems to be less talk about *dopamine,* which is responsible for emotional balance and pleasure. Increased levels of dopamine are experienced with sex and use of stimulants. *Norepinephrine* is known for promoting drive and motivation. *Acetylcholine,* another neurotransmitter, promotes memory, attention, and sleep—all vital during the transition into menopause. As estrogen drops in perimenopause, the balance of neurotransmitters in the brain becomes challenged; without a balance, depression is more likely. *Selective serotonin reuptake inhibitors* (SSRIs), the newest generation of antidepressants, have provided a much-needed option for care of the client with depression. A major scientific contribution in the mental health community, SSRIs have fewer difficult side effects, quicker onset of action, and the ability to provide relief from the dark side of depression. Some brand names are Prozac, Paxil, Zoloft, Lexapro, and Celexa. Simply put, SSRIs inhibit the reuptake or metabolization of serotonin so that more is available in the brain to keep the tender balance.

My rule of thumb for clients who have experienced periods of depression at any junction in life is to pay attention to your moods. You are more likely to dip into the pit of depression when multiple stressors are encountered, a major loss occurs, or too many challenges pile up all at once. But it becomes my job to help clients uncover their early warning signals and thus be better prepared. Early warning signals of depression could be loss of interest in those activities that usually bring you joy, sleeping more, sleeping less than your norm, being more easily frustrated, eating less, using comfort foods more often and in excess, and avoiding people and social activities. In therapy sessions, I invite my clients to write on one side of a colored index card the early warning signals of depression and on the opposite side list the coping skills in their repertoire.

Suzie, a recent client, was referred because of perimenopausal symptoms of hot flashes, sleep cycle dysfunction, decreased libido, loss of energy, and irritability with her husband and sons. An attractive, smiling woman entered the office that sunny July day. At first, I wondered about the referral. Suzie seemed to have life in a neat package. She had her own business, a loving husband, two vivacious boys, and lovely home. "I just can not keep up this pace. Everyone wants something from me—my time, my organizational skills, my energy, and of course my attention. My husband doesn't have a clue how unhappy I am. I do not like the woman I have turned into." Suzie had begun avoiding friends and calls from family members, going back to bed when she got the boys off to school, and having frequent headaches. Sitting in session, she also realized the "loss of self"—what happened to that vivacious woman ready to set the world on fire? Identifying the early warning signals for her mild depression assisted in developing the next steps for a plan to prevent her mild depression from turning into a major depression. Since this was her first known depressive episode, the importance of successful interventions and resolution of her symptoms became our goal. Coping skills appeared to have been lost in her juggling multiple roles and agendas. Going back into her early years to revisit coping techniques, she discovered the joy of listening to music, exercise, talking to supportive people, tennis, gardening, and dance, all activities known to replenish her energy and spirit. With her colored index card in her wallet and a few additional sessions to discuss integrating them into her life, we could then tackle the other perimenopausal issues bringing her into treatment.

An important message for Suzie regarding depression is this: do not let five days go by plagued by your early warning signals and engage your coping skills. In fact, she may need to execute two or three for relief of symptoms. If two weeks of depressed mood persist even with the use of copers, make an appointment with your therapist or provider and get into the office. And listen to family members; they may see some signals before you do.

There is no blood test for diagnosing depression. Future research may unlock profiles for a variety of types of depression and subsequent treatments along with the research of brain scans and imaging in today's forefront. Various types of depression and a list of symptoms provide a deeper understanding of this plaguing mood state.

Types of Depression

Major or Clinical Depression
Chronic feelings of sadness, hopelessness, and apathy that are out of proportion to life's events. Diagnosis depends on the presence of five or more symptoms (listed next) that have persisted for at least two weeks and that interfere with your function at home or work or socially.

Mild Depression
Fewer symptoms with less disruption in life; do not ignore the condition, especially if daily function is impaired or an episode previously occurred.

Moderate Depression
A significant number of symptoms exist and greatly affect daily function.

Severe Depression
Function in most areas of life—home, work, and social—are impaired with all or most of the symptoms listed present.

Seasonal Affective Disorder (SAD)
A pattern persists for at least two years of cyclic sadness and depressive symptoms that worsen during a particular time of year or when there is less sunlight. Remission occurs when sunlight returns. Winter months seem to accelerate seasonal affective disorder with resolution in spring.

Symptoms of Depression

For a diagnosis of depression, five or more of the following symptoms must be present and persist for most of a two-week period (including one of the first two):

- Persistent sad mood
- Loss of interest or pleasure with activities you previously enjoyed
- Loss of energy
- Sleep cycle dysfunction—difficulty falling asleep, early morning awakening, or oversleeping
- Appetite changes and weight changes
- Sense of worthlessness
- Difficulty making decisions
- Physical agitation or retarded movements
- Thoughts of death or suicide

TREATMENT OPTIONS

Treatment options for depression vary with the type of depression and therapist preference. Psychotherapy sometimes referred to as "talk therapy" is the most common form of intervention for mild to moderate depression. Psychotherapy is a structured encounter between client and therapist employing communication and a therapeutic relationship to uncover conflicted issues, increase awareness, and cope better with problems of life. Psychoanalysis the first specific school of psychotherapy began in the nineteenth century with Sigmund Freud's contributions. Since then, a multitude of theorists and approaches developed for client treatment. Most clinicians begin the process with a general client history and in-depth assessment of the presenting issue. Referrals often provide a physical history and laboratory results in an effort to rule out physiological problems. This menopausal era of hormonal flux can often be associated with organ dysfunction, so it is critical to rule out physiological issues from depressive profiles. Psychotherapy can be for the individual, couples, or the family system to assist in resolving troubled relationships, personal traumas, family crises, or transitional states.

Cognitive-behavioral therapy (CBT) has become a standard for treating depression. It helps individuals examine thinking and behaviors in response to situations they encounter. Simply put, the client is encouraged to examine the way she thinks—what messages automatically flow in her mind. Thus, it could be said that "what you think predicts what you feel, and thinking and feeling move you to action or a behavior." Such therapy invites the client to be more flexible and to confront negative cognitions, assumptions, beliefs, and behaviors. Albert Ellis and Aaron Beck were early pioneers in this therapeutic modality. In more than 400 studies, CBT has proven to be an effective process in reducing symptoms and preventing relapse for clients with depression. In fact, in 2000, a large-scale study demonstrated higher results of response and remission when a form of CBT and an antidepressant were combined than when either modality was used alone.[8] The cognitive distortions resulting from negative thinking patterns are challenged with this process and provide an opportunity for individuals to gain greater control over life by correcting the distortions and restructuring a new positive cognition.

Moderate or severe depression responds most effectively to an approach combining psychotherapy with medication. This combination has been proven to have fewer recurrences over a three-year period than those receiving one or the other, according to a National Institute of Mental Health study.[9]

Light therapy for seasonal affective disorders is an accepted treatment modality. The clinician prescribes use of a "light box" once to several times a day, for 15 minutes to an hour, depending on severity of symptoms. The intensity of the light exposure assists many patients to feel better in one to two weeks. Often a prescription can help with insurance reimbursement for the light box, which can cost up to $200.

Now a few words about the benefits of *exercise*, which boosts the level of neurotransmitters in the brain, those chemicals linked to mood. Far too many women are unaware of the ability to reduce and manage their depressive symptoms with consistent exercise. In addition, endorphins, the body's natural narcotic, are released with vigorous exercise. We are not talking about hours in the gym, running miles every day, or even training programs for a marathon, though these are options to improve health and well-being. I am encouraging walking—a brisk walk starting with 10 minutes three times a week and progressing to 30 minutes every day or five times a week.

Two therapeutic modalities for medication-resistant depressed patients are *electroconvulsive therapy* and *vagus nerve stimulation.* Electroconvulsive therapy for the treatment of resistive depression has long been an option. I remember assisting psychiatrists with the procedure in the mid-1970s on a psychiatric unit in a local general hospital. Although it remains an option today, there are downsides to its use. Patients usually experience memory loss and cognitive problems. They may resolve quickly but not always, and in some cases periods of memory are lost forever. Electroconvulsive therapy is not a permanent resolution to depression, resulting in several rounds of treatment with relapse potential. Vagus nerve stimulation, a new approach, began for use with patients having drug-resistant epilepsy. For the patient with medication-resistant depression, a pacemaker-like device is surgically attached to the left vagus nerve in the neck to stimulate mood centers. One pilot study showed that about one-third of patients had a 50 percent decrease in their depression. The downside is that it can take up to one year for optimal results to be achieved.

Each modality mentioned brings benefits to an individual suffering from depression. Women experiencing pronounced and persistent mood states do not have to struggle alone through them. You do have options. Talk to your health care provider when your mood state does not improve after attempts to resolve the sad feelings or after two weeks of struggle. I am glad to say that the stigma associated with mental illness has lessened, and the wise woman of this generation is not afraid to reach out for professional help.

PRESCRIPTIVE INTERVENTIONS

Antidepressant medications work by slowing the removal of certain chemicals from the brain. These chemicals are called neurotransmitters, the most common being serotonin and norepinephrine. Neurotransmitters are needed for normal brain function and are involved in the control of mood and other functions, such as eating, sleeping, experiencing pain, and thinking. Antidepressants make these natural chemicals more available to the brain, restore the chemical balance, and relieve the symptoms of depression. Helping to reduce the extreme sadness, hopelessness, and lack of interest in life that people with depression face is a major benefit of antidepressant treatment.

Antidepressants are typically taken for six to nine months and in some cases longer, depending on the patient's history and response to medications. The general rule is one year because of relapse potential. Clients with three or more episodes of depression are often encouraged to remain on medications to lessen the chance of another debilitating depression. Studies have reported that 80 percent of depressed clients respond to medication therapy. During the prescriptive phase of treatment, several medications may need to be tried before finding one that works for you. It is important not to abandon a medication prematurely; give it a four- to six-week trial before moving on. Too many of my clients seeking the magic pill lose interest after one or two weeks of a medication trial even after I have informed them it is trial and error at this point in psychopharmacology. The *New England Journal of Medicine* found that one out of every three or four clients may need to change to another prescription or add an adjunctive medication to obtain relief of symptoms. And like most medications, antidepressants can cause adverse reactions. Much depends on your body and the medication chosen. Talk to your health care provider if adverse reactions are bothersome.

Tricyclics, the original or first generation of antidepressants, act on serotonin, norepinephrine, and other chemicals in the body. Tricyclic medications include Elavil (amitriptyline), Norpramine (desipramine), Tofranil (imipramine), Aventyl, and Pamelor (nortriptyline). Common adverse reactions are dry mouth, blurred vision, constipation, difficulty urinating, worsening of glaucoma, tiredness, impaired thinking, and, for some, effects on blood pressure and heart rate. The fact that this group of medications acts on other chemicals in the body may be responsible for the varied and often disruptive adverse effects on the patient.

The SSRIs are the second generation of antidepressants and are more widely used because of their less severe adverse reactions, quicker onset, and effectiveness in resolving disturbing symptoms of depression. Included in this category are Lexapro (escitalopram), Celexa (citalopram), Prozac (fluoxetine), Paxil (paroxetine), and Zoloft (sertraline). Lexapro is noted to be fast acting. Prozac and Paxil have been effective in reducing hot flashes in some women yet cause hot flashes in others. Adverse reactions seen with this category are dry mouth, nausea, nervousness, insomnia, headache, skin rashes, weight gain, and weight loss. Sexual problems found with this medication group relate to difficulty reaching orgasm. Women already struggling with a low or slowed sexual response should be aware of this complication. Some women report a resolution of the problem after a few months of use, while others are prescribed another antidepressant, Wellbutrin, in an attempt to counteract the orgasmic retardation.

Serotonin-norepinephrine reuptake inhibitors (SNRIs) have gained popularity in the past few years since they work on serotonin and norepinephrine in the brain. Effexor (venlafxine) and Cymbalta (duloxetine) are in this category. Adverse reactions include sleepiness, dizziness, constipation, and sexual dysfunction. This category becomes the second group used in medication trials when women fail SSRI trials. Cymbalta is also prescribed for peripheral neuropathic pain from diabetes and fibromyalgia. Wellbutrin (bupropion) is in a different category because of its action sites. Thus, the versatility of Wellbutrin is seen for relief of depression, sexual side effects of antidepressants, as an adjunctive medication, and even restless legs syndrome.

The last category reviewed, monoamine oxidase inhibitors (MAOIs), were introduced in the 1950s. These work to increase the functioning of both serotonin and norepinephrine in the brain. Nardil (phenelzine) and Parnate (tranylcypromine) are the most common MAOIs utilized today. The strict dietary and alcohol restrictions, drug interactions, and adverse reactions have limited the prescriptive use of this category. Restrictions include aged foods, red wine, soy sauce, and certain cheeses. A new MAOI patch (transdermal selegiline) does not have the same restrictions and holds new opportunities for care of the depressed patient.

ANXIETY DISORDERS

Research studies provide evidence that *anxiety* affects twice as many women as men. Feeling anxious because of a particular situation, such as making a presentation at work or church, differs from an *anxiety disorder,* in which you experience an exaggerated response to an event or challenge you are facing. Studies of younger women with panic attacks have established that their anxiety is greater around the time of their menstrual cycle. These young women may be at a greater risk for an anxiety disorder around perimenopause because of hormonal fluctuations. An anxiety disorder is caused by a biochemical imbalance triggering the "fight-or-flight" response of the body: pounding heart, difficulty breathing, and sweating. Following are brief descriptions of anxiety disorders.

Generalized anxiety disorder is excessive, uncontrollable, and often irrational worry about everyday things that is out of proportion to the actual source of worry. The worried state continues for more days than not and over at least a six-month period. Everyday concerns could be related to finances, health, family matters, or work. Treatment options include psychotherapy, SSRI or SNRI medication, benzodiazepines, kava (an herb), and CBT.

Social anxiety disorder is an experience of fear, apprehension, or worry regarding social situations along with a fear of embarrassment or humiliation by others. Physical symptoms include excessive blushing, sweating, trembling, palpitations, nausea, and stammering. Treatment options include psychotherapy, SSRI or SNRI medication, and CBT.

Panic disorder is a condition characterized by recurring panic attacks in combination with behavioral changes or at least a month of ongoing worry about having another attack. Panic attacks can last 10 minutes or be as short as one to five minutes in length. *Panic attacks* are described as having rapid heartbeat, perspiration, dizziness, difficulty breathing, or trembling with a sense of uncontrollable fear. If left untreated, panic disorders can worsen and cause upheaval in the person's life, sometimes leading to agoraphobia, or the inability to leave one's home. These disturbing symptoms can lead one to believe that they are having a life-threatening illness. Many emergency room visits and medical testing may occur before a diagnosis and treatment plan are in place. Again, psychotherapy, medications, and CBT are options for treatment.

Phobias are irrational, intense, persistent fears of certain situations, objects, activities, or persons. The National Institute of Mental Health found that between 8.7 and 18.1 percent of Americans suffer from phobias. Cognitive-behavioral therapy is beneficial along with desensitization exercises to deal with the specific fear, such as a fear of flying, snakes, spiders, or social situations.

Obsessive-compulsive disorder (OCD) is characterized by an individual's obsessive, distressing, intrusive thoughts and related compulsions (tasks or rituals) that attempt to neutralize the obsession. Debate continues whether OCD is a psychological disorder or is caused by abnormalities in the brain. It is typically treated with behavioral therapy, CBT, medication, or a combination of the three.

Posttraumatic stress disorder (PTSD) is another anxiety disorder that can develop after exposure to a terrifying event or physical harm that occurred or was threatened. Persistent symptoms of arousal, hypervigilance, avoidance, and the reexperiencing of the event for more than one month make up the diagnosis of PTSD. Traumatic experiences include a serious accident, medical complications, physical assault or threat, sexual assault, natural disasters, warfare, and, most recently, the trauma of cancer survivors. Early intervention after a traumatic incident, known as critical incident stress management, is often used to reduce the effects of trauma. Combination therapy of psychotherapy, CBT, exposure therapy, medication, and eye movement desensitization and reprocessing (EMDR) are all beneficial in helping the client in moving beyond the traumatic event.

In summary, let me offer an observation: the woman in menopausal transition may find herself struggling with depressive symptoms. Do not struggle for long or too hard, as options are available. Begin by confronting your cognitions: are your thoughts negative and sabotaging your own success? Reframe that mental picture, think from a positive position, and use affirmations as antidotes for negative thinking. What lifestyle adjustments can be added to move past the dark side of depression? Coping skills, diet, exercise, and prayer are wonderful options. Many times the strategies used in therapy help women redefine their thinking, make adjustments in lifestyle, and add new coping skills. So do not underestimate your abilities—with a little guidance.

STRESS

To present a full picture of emotional well-being, we need to direct some attention to stress. *Stress* comes in all shapes, sizes, and intensity. The positive impact of stress moves you to complete a task or project or even to finish those last 10 minutes on the treadmill. Persistent stress that is not resolved by coping or adaptation can lead to escape (anxiety) or withdrawal (depression) behaviors. Protracted stress wears out your immune system. Your health depends on how you manage stress in everyday life.

There are three types of stress:

> *"Everyday life" stress*—The roles you juggle being a wife, mother, daughter, friend, homemaker, businesswoman, nurse, or teacher. You cannot totally eliminate or ignore it, but how you attend to this type of stress or adapt to it determines your resilience.

"Can't get away from it" stress—This is more destructive than day-to-day stress. It wears away your well-being. The holiday plans you do not have the energy to address, tires wearing out on your daughter's car, and a project at work that awakens you at 2:00 in the morning are good examples of this type of stress.

"Major life events" stress—Examples are chronic illness, children leaving home, divorce, death of a family member, or even the arrival of a new grandchild. Over time, these bring more intensity to your adaptation, and studies have proven that having two or more major life events can challenge even the most capable person.

Managing stress well creates a sense of empowerment. Stress, like conflict, is inevitable; the fight-or-flight response of stress may challenge the body's homeostasis and increase blood pressure, accelerate heart rate, increase concentration, and release stress hormones from the hypothalamic-pituitary-adrenal (HPA) axis. When too much stress occurs because of an accident; an illness such as an ulcer, a heart attack, or cancer; or the constant worry of an anxiety disorder, the HPA axis becomes overworked and exhausted, ultimately damaging tissues, cells, and organs in the body.

Internal threats, external threats, and life's challenges began in childhood. As an adult, the anger, perhaps your rebellion of childhood, was, it is hoped, replaced with a new mind-set, coping skills, and support networks. What are your initial thoughts and reactions when challenged or stressed by life? Do you reach inside and reframe the issue? Do you break it into small pieces or steps so as not to overwhelm yourself? Does that supportive friend enter your mind as a resource to bounce ideas off or just to vent? Maybe on the way home, you make a date for yourself at the gym; this is an ideal way to manage stress. Some people go toward comfort foods—not an entirely bad idea, but be cautious that it doesn't become your only or favorite strategy. Deep breathing, walking outside, stretching, head rolls, shoulder shrugs, and visualizing a peaceful place are tangible options to employ. The next chapter goes into more depth as we look at coping skills and options for well-being. Resilience, that internal armor you wear to strengthen your resolve, helps you weather those emotional hurricanes and help you do more than just survive; with resilience as a traveling companion, you *thrive*. Turn to chapter 7 and commit to not only examining the options for resilience but also selecting two or perhaps three new skills for the next year.

Chapter Seven

COMPLEMENTARY AND ALTERNATIVE STRATEGIES FOR THE MIDLIFE WOMAN

When so rich a harvest is before us, why do we not gather it? All is in our hands if we will but use it.

—Elizabeth Seton

In the previous chapter, "emotional well-being for the seasoned woman" was described with techniques to unearth a view of the past, models to examine options for the future, and emotional conditions like depression, anxiety, and stress that can challenge even the most resilient woman. This chapter provides many options for coping with the body's natural evolution into menopause. The "seasoned woman" as identified by Gail Sheehy has determination and a conviction to use her lived experiences to maximize the menopause journey. "Lived experiences" are those health events, relationship encounters, and environmental incidents that order a person's life and shape a person's perspective. What health initiatives produced positive benefits in the past? What supplements or dietary aids make up the daily regime? In my office setting, newspaper articles, magazine proclamations, morning news programs, and a friend's recommendation of new menopause therapies often become the discourse during the interview with a new client. Let me share some of the many areas discussed by today's woman in and out of the therapist's office.

Before addressing the strategies, let's delve into coping skills. I alluded to copers in the previous chapter and identified a few, such as exercise, talking to a supportive person, and relaxation exercises. I also challenged you to identify coping skills that warranted a deep look and asked you to select two or three for the upcoming year to enhance your current degree of resilience. So what is a coping skill, and how do you assess the copers you currently possess to determine their effectiveness? Coping skills are behavioral tools used to overcome an adversity or stressor. Every person possesses several negative and several positive copers. A negative coper could be alcohol, smoking, overeating to deal with the bombardment of stress, divorce, illness, or other upsetting life factors. I would suggest two primary styles to assist you in coping with stress: action-based coping and emotion-based coping.

TWO PRIMARY STYLES TO COPE WITH STRESS

Action-based coping moves an individual to deal "directly" with the problem that is causing the stress. Hot flashes and sleep deprivation are causing Mary physical and emotional distress. She made an appointment with her nurse-midwife to review her options and reduce the symptom discomfort of her menopause transition.

Emotion-based coping skills reduce the stress without addressing the source. Mary's positive coping led her to call a close friend and share how her perimenopausal symptoms were disrupting her life. She felt better, but she has not ultimately solved the problem. After the phone call, her stress may be at a manageable level and move her to an action-based approach, such as making another call or scheduling an appointment to see her midwife, thus directly dealing with the problem.

Coping techniques for today's busy woman are given in Appendix A. This exercise is a standard in my private practice for depressed, anxious, overwhelmed women. Frequently, when stress overwhelms one's world, even the previous effective techniques to reduce stress are forgotten or the motivation to revisit them is absent. Producing the exercise as a homework activity can be enlightening. I have divided the techniques into six categories: diversions, mental, relationship, physical, interpersonal, and spiritual. An individual takes the exercise home and circles current negative copers in use first and then the positive copers utilized. The challenge becomes identifying two or three new strategies and putting them into the daily life routine. Depressed or overwhelmed people rarely have the psychic energy to think up new copers much less the motivation to proceed to action.

My general rule of thumb regarding coping skills is that each one of us is compelled to identify five coping strategies from a variety of settings, collect them on an index card and put it in your wallet, tape them to the inside of a cupboard in your bathroom, and make them readily available at your fingertips. You never know when the stress of everyday living might pile up and you lose sight of well-being. Having five dependable coping strategies available enhances your ability to dig out of a difficult time. My all-time favorites are journaling, music, exercise, talking to someone supportive, and reframing issues into positive affirmations. You can see that some of these are action oriented, others more an internal dialogue. In fact, there have been times when engaging one did not relieve pressure—another reason you need a variety of strategies. Making this part of the therapy process for my clients seems to provide the buy-in to get things started. My challenge to you: do not end this chapter without doing this exercise, then share it with a friend or loved one.

One weekend before returning to the computer to work on this chapter, I was reading the Sunday paper with my husband, our Sunday ritual with coffee in hand. In the *Parade* magazine section, up pops an article: "How Stress Makes You Flabby" by Michael O'Shea. He cited a study by Dr. Zofia Zukowska, the senior author, of Georgetown University Medical Center. The study suggests a physiological reason that people gain weight under stress. Dr. Zukowska says, "Researchers suspect that stress and diet stimulate an enzyme present in particularly high amounts in the abdominal fat." And where do most peri- and postmenopausal women complain of a fat buildup? The belly. So even if your calorie intake doesn't go up during stressful times, the enzyme released because of your stress will promote fat deposits in the stomach. Additionally, "the most dangerous place for fat to end up is in the abdomen since it increases the risk for heart disease, hypertension and diabetes," states O'Shea. Dr. Zukowska remarks, "Paying attention to the fact that stress may amplify weight gain means it's important to include relaxation therapy as part of any weight-loss program. Exercise remains one of the most effective antidotes, because it lowers stress hormones. Even a 15-minute walk can help break the cycle."[1] Incorporating some of the previously cited coping skills and options available in the next section promotes well-being, stress reduction, and, for those weight-conscious glamorous seasoned women, a decrease of abdominal fat. Sign me up for yoga, Pilates, and a brisk 15-minute walk.

COMPLEMENTARY AND ALTERNATIVE MEDICINE

Complementary and alternative medicine (CAM) provide additional healing philosophies, therapies, and approaches beyond the discussion in many conventional medicine offices in this country. However, the majority of women entering menopause either have considered these many approaches or are utilizing them and wonder how effective they are for menopause intervention. Complementary therapies represent those strategies used in addition to conventional treatment. Alternative approaches are utilized instead of conventional treatment. In 2002, a national representative sample of women reported that 45 percent of respondents ages 45 to 57 used CAM practices in the past 12 months. Only 3 percent mentioned using CAM specifically to treat menopause or menopausal symptoms. Canadian researchers state in a 2003 study that some 20 percent of Canadians age 12 and older have consulted an alternative care provider in the past year and that 70 percent of Canadian citizens use "natural health products," including herbal products, vitamins and mineral supplements, and homeopathic medications as well as traditional medicine.[2] In the Study of Women's Health Across the Nation (SWAN), a 10-year longitudinal trial of several ethnic groups of U.S. women, a recent report established more than one-half of women used some type of CAM.[3] Given the large proportion of midlife women who use CAM and the potential for interactions with prescribed medications, women and health care providers need to discuss which interventions are part of a daily routine and review current medication profiles.

My insight regarding clients involved in CAM therapies is that they have chosen to do so because of their value system, their beliefs, or the benefits noted. And then some women turn to these modalities after frustration and dissatisfaction with Western medicine. Often the waiting period for an appointment with a health care provider is too long. Adverse reactions to medications can be daunting, or a "grin-and-bear-it" approach for today's assertive woman is just not part of her health care vocabulary. Another factor ever present in the makeup of this modern woman is a "holistic" philosophy toward health and self-care. A holistic mind-set promotes positive health habits, a responsibility to take part in the decision making for one's health and healing. All these components lead women to seek other options in the CAM therapy continuum. The hallmark of a competent and empathetic clinician is supporting women where they are in their process, accepting their need for some control during a perplexing life cycle, and remaining nonjudgmental as they problem solve treatment options.

In 1998, the U.S. Congress established the National Center for Complementary and Alternative Medicine (NCCAM) at the National Institutes of Health to stimulate, develop, and support research on CAM therapies to benefit the public. The NCCAM evaluates the safety and effectiveness of CAM modalities, trains CAM researchers, and produces reliable information for dissemination to citizens. A clearinghouse of recent research, clinical trials, and training options and a popular section with updates on treatments and herbal advances can be found at http:/nccam.nih.gov.

The NCCAM divides CAM therapies into five categories: (1) alternative medical systems, (2) mind–body medicine, (3) manipulative and body-based methods, (4) energy medicine, and (5) biologically based treatment. A brief account of some of the more popular modalities is identified here. As you review this section, I ask you to consider two new options to integrate into your day-to-day life for the next six months. Adding complementary and therapeutic endeavors benefits the mind and body of today's seasoned woman and solidifies your status as a "seasoned siren."

Alternative medical systems include traditional Chinese medicine, acupuncture, Ayurveda medicine, homeopathic medicine, and naturopathic medicine. *Traditional Chinese medicine* establishes the need for balance between the two opposing forces of yin and yang. Yin represents the cold, slow, or passive component, while Yang represents the hot, excited, or active component of the body. Acupuncture, herbal intervention, tai chi, and oriental massage move the body back into harmony thus removing the blockage of qi (pronounced "chee," meaning vital energy).

Traditional Chinese medicine practitioners often treat women with menopause utilizing *acupuncture* procedures. Acupuncture can be traced back at least 2,500 years. It wasn't until President Richard Nixon's trip to China in 1972 that an explosion of curiosity regarding acupuncture and then augmentation into Western medicine took place. Acupuncture involves stimulation of anatomic points in the body, for therapeutic purposes, usually by puncturing the skin with a needle. The Food and Drug Administration (FDA) approved the use of acupuncture needles by licensed practitioners in 1996. A rich list of ailments aided by the use of acupuncture include energy disturbances, pain relief, emotional dysfunctions, addictions, relief of nausea and vomiting for chemotherapy and surgery, prevention of illness, and induction of analgesia. Clinical trials in 2006 and 2007 found acupuncture to significantly reduce the severity of nighttime hot flashes but not necessarily their frequency.[4] Yet anecdotal reports from clinicians and clients pepper magazines and books regarding the alleviation of perplexing symptoms through the use of acupuncture.

Tai chi, derived from Chinese medicine, proposes that a combination of exercise and energy work can stimulate the flow of chi, or life energy. The slow, continuous, controlled movements resemble a graceful dance. Proven benefits for the woman with arthritis and improved coordination, reduction in falls, and reduction of stress add to the attraction of this modality for the menopausal woman.

Ayurveda is India's traditional system of medicine. Equal emphasis is placed on body, mind, and spirit with efforts to restore harmony and balance within the individual. Ayurveda treatments include controlled breathing, massage, meditation, exercise, diet, and herbs. This modality has risen to the forefront because of the popular writings of Deepak Chopra.

Homeopathic medicine was developed in the late eighteenth century by Samuel Hahnemann. Until the early 1900s, homeopathy was not commonly practiced in the United States. Western medicine discredited the treatment approach, stating that it was not based on scientific models and not effective. Yet in recent years, the popularity has risen again in the CAM community.

Focus for this modality is on the links between the client's physical, emotional, and mental systems. Minute doses of specially prepared plant extracts and minerals are used to stimulate the body's healing processes. Three of the most common remedies for the peri- and postmenopausal woman are lachesis (derived from venom of the South American bushmaster snake, pulsatilla (derived from the wildflower *Anemone pulsatilla*), and sepia (derived from cuttlefish ink).[5]

The foundation of *naturopathic medicine* emphasizes health restoration rather than disease treatment. Naturopathic physicians often practice as primary care providers in communities. They provide a multitude of healing practices, including acupuncture, exercise, diet, nutrition, herbal medicine, and spinal and soft tissue manipulation to assist the body's natural healing processes.

Mind–body medicine supports the interaction among the brain, mind, body, and behavior to affect one's health. In 2002, mind–body techniques, including relaxation techniques, meditation, guided imagery, yoga, biofeedback, and hypnosis, were used by about 17 percent of the adult U.S. population. Mind–body interventions constitute a major portion of the overall use of CAM by the public. Clinical evidence supports the effectiveness of mind–body interventions used in addition to conventional medicine to improve quality of life and reduce anxiety and pain. Studies at Yale and Rutgers universities by Ellen Idler, PhD, and Stanislav Kasi, PhD, revealed that the self-image toward health and well-being is a significant predictor of future health conditions.[6] For the peri- and postmenopausal woman, this research substantiates the need to continue building a strong and vibrant self-image and relationship to health. Embracing techniques from the mind–body continuum and practicing them on a consistent basis enhances future health for those decades beyond the menopause transition. In my private practice, I continue to challenge the overwhelmed newly identified perimenopausal woman to strengthen her self-image and accept this process as temporary, with interval dips into the pool of symptoms and the use of therapeutic techniques to restore health and well-being.

Relaxation techniques make up a group of behavioral and therapeutic approaches within the family of mind–body medicine. As a clinician and perimenopausal woman, this group of techniques is rich with possibilities and restorative properties. The *relaxation response* is a state of deep relaxation that physiologically lowers heart and breathing rates, reduces muscle tension, and decreases metabolic activity. When utilized regularly over time, the relaxation response can decrease hot flashes in the perimenopausal woman and assist her with managing stress in everyday life. The SWAN study followed more than 3,300 women through their perimenopausal years and discovered that when meditation, yoga, and relaxation are integrated into daily life, there is a reduction in the severity of hot flashes.

In the 1970s, Herbert Benson, a Harvard Medical School cardiologist, reported his research on the relaxation response, and since then meditation and relaxation techniques have found their way into many a clinician's office.[7] The process of relaxation encompasses repetitive focus on a word, sound, prayer, phrase, body sensation, or muscular activity and, second, a passive attitude, banishing intruding thoughts while remaining focused on the original word or sound. Teaching the relaxation response to women in the office, I invite the pupil to think of the fall season and leaves descending from the trees. The leaf drifts slowly through the air currents until it gently rests on the ground. Their awareness is much like the leaf; it drifts out of the day's schedule, out of the preceding activity, and into this moment, allowing any intrusive thoughts to be gently pushed aside and instead surrendering to the moment of "peace" while slowly following my count from 10 to 1. As the number 1 is encountered, the pupil imagines the leaf resting quietly on the ground and the body and mind becoming calm, peaceful, tranquil, and relaxed. On completing the guided relaxation exercise, I share a CD with the narrative the pupil has just experienced as the homework assignment. Several clients struggling with nighttime hot flashes and insomnia have decreased the awakening period and the intensity of hot flashing by employing the CD at that time.

Relaxation strategies vary from the previously guided activity to techniques such as relaxing each part of the body; visualization techniques with a focus on a scene at the mountains, ocean, or other peaceful places; the use of music with environmental scenes; or even a hot bath with lavender and chamomile oils.

Another intervention needing to be mentioned for its benefits is *meditation*. Meditation is self-directed practice for relaxing the body and calming the mind. The goal of mindfulness meditation asks the participant to move into a nonjudgmental awareness of body sensations and mental activities and "be" in the present moment. One well-liked form of meditation is *Transcendental Meditation*, which centers on a "suitable" sound or thought (the mantra) without attempting to actively concentrate on the sound or thought. My initial introduction to TM was in the mid-1970s. I was completing nursing school in Dallas, Texas, and preparing to take the licensing board. What a valuable technique to promote centering one's mind, removing the debris from the day and applying a focus to breathing and my mantra. Not only did I pass the nursing boards, but TM became a frequent ally in graduate school at Boston University a few years later.

Yoga, a favorite refueling technique of mine, is another component within the mind–body category. The disciplines of yoga had their origins in India with a connection to religious beliefs and practices. Within the practice of yoga, there exist a variety of branches. In the Western world, hatha yoga is the better known with its asanas (postures) and the meditative element to purify mind, spirit, and body. Documentation and anecdotal notes reflect the benefits of yoga for the menopausal woman. Books, articles, exercise DVDs, and classes are abundant to help women bring energy and balance into their lives. And what menopausal woman in the transition couldn't use a little energy and balance? Yoga stretches and exercises promote better blood circulation and oxygenation to all cells and tissues. This helps optimize the function of the endocrine glands (which are already taking a beating), the reproductive tract, the digestive tract, the nervous system, and other organs stressed during menopause.

I cannot discuss the benefits of yoga and not include *Pilates* as another valuable practice for women in transition. But did you know the origins of Pilates? Joseph Pilates developed the physical fitness system of Pilates during World War I to improve the rehabilitation program for returning veterans. Strengthening, stretching, and stabilizing key muscles is the foundation of this method. Centering the body and mind through controlled breathing, stretching, and fundamental movements with a focus on the "powerhouse," or "core" (abdomen, lower back, hips, and buttocks), of the body then become the elements of this successful method for the menopausal woman.

Another mind-body exercise—Nia—is a transformational movement that draws from dance arts, martial arts, and healing arts. It aids in strengthening muscles, weight loss, calms the mind and relieves tension. And yet, it was the dance movements that sold me. Nia invites a connection of the sensual spirit with body movement and music that unleashes a grace awareness of your body that basic dance just cannot do. Find a Nia teacher in your area and try it just once, their web site is www.NiaNow.com. The sensual you will be awakened.

Many menopausal and postmenopausal women are frustrated by symptoms of irritability, hot flashes, and weight gain, especially around the midsection. One study conducted in the summer of 2006 concluded that vigorous physical activity significantly reduces body fat and waist size. The bottom line is that although our bodies change with age, we have more control over the end result. With Pilates and yoga, women can notice an improvement in body toning, range of motion, flexibility in the hips shoulders, and less overall back pain. The choice is yours: exercise and specific techniques such as yoga and Pilates with a healthy diet are options for a more vital you in the upcoming decades of good living.

Deep breathing exercises offer another approach to reduce anxiety and pain. The brief method of deep breathing is versatile in that it can be done at work, while riding home in traffic, or during the unraveling of a conflict or any tense moment. Deep breathing involves taking several deep breaths, holding them for five seconds, and then exhaling slowly.

Biofeedback techniques use monitoring instruments used to measure bodily processes such as blood pressure, heart rate, skin temperature, sweating, and muscle tension and relay the information directly to the individual to raise her awareness and conscious control of the activity. Biofeedback has been used with much success to control hot flashes. Studies also report a reduction of the frequency of incontinence episodes for women trained with bladder-sphincter biofeedback techniques. Dannecker's 2005 study of biofeedback-assisted pelvic-floor-muscle training showed the effectiveness in treating stress urinary or mixed incontinence.[8] Physical therapy colleagues utilize biofeedback and pelvic-floor strengthening exercise for many of the clients I see with vulvadynia and vaginismus, an involuntary constriction of the vaginal muscles that prevents sexual intercourse. Small biofeedback machines are available for home use. The collaborative approach between sex therapists and physical therapists to assist women with these two very painful and sexually debilitating experiences is certainly enhanced with biofeedback.

Manipulative and body-based methods within the CAM family were developed through the practice of manipulation or movement of body structures and systems to restore health. Chiropractors focus on the structure of the spine and its function while manipulating body parts to maximize health. Chiropractors are licensed by states, and most insurance companies reimburse their treatments.

Reflexology is a therapeutic method of relieving pain by stimulating predefined pressure points on the feet and hands. The controlled pressure alleviates the discomfort. Reflexology is also effective for promoting good health and relief of stress. The pressure-point mapping that is utilized connects directly to the nervous system and affects bodily organs and glands. One exercise included in either the Sexplore Weekend Retreats for couples that I facilitate or the couples sessions to rebuild trust are hand and foot massage utilizing a reflexology map.

Energy medicine focuses on energy fields originating in the body. Two modes highlighted in this section are Reiki and Healing Touch. *Reiki,* the Japanese word representing universal life energy, is based on channeling "healing energy" through the practitioner's palms to bring about healing. In this mode, the healing comes from the universe not the therapist; in *Healing Touch,* the healing force, or "laying-on of hands," comes from the therapist and balancing the body's energy forces.

Biologically based treatments overlap with conventional Western medicine. Examples are special diet therapies to prevent illness and to promote health: Atkins, South Beach, Zone, Ornish, and Pritikin diet plans, to name a few. Herbal and botanical therapies have increased their market share for the perimenopausal and menopausal woman since the early termination of the estrogen and progestin arm of the Women's Health Initiative.

A French chemist, Rene Maurice Gattefosse, was the first to use the word *aromatherapy* in the 1920s after an accident in his perfume laboratory. Lavender oil was birthed that day for its surprising pain relief and speed in burn healing. Aromatherapy is the use of essential oils from plants to purposefully affect a person's mood or health. Application modes include aerial diffusion, direct inhalation, topical application, or use in the mouth, rectum, and vagina. In France, essential oils are incorporated into mainstream medicine. In our Western culture, they seem to be more of an augmentation to medical practice.

Botanical treatments administer complex mixtures of preparations made from the whole plant or plant part, such as root, leaves, gum, resin, or essential oil. A medicinal herb is a plant or plant part that produces and contains chemical substances that act on the body. *Herbal therapies* can be given in a variety of ways:

- Essential oils (highly concentrated)
- Dried extracts
- Diluted preparations
- Tinctures and fluid extracts from plants
- Tea infusions, steeped but not boiled

Herbal drugs established their presence since the 1970s with the advent of over-the-counter (OTC) tablets, capsules, and extracts. However, one issue that perplexes consumers and clinicians alike is the quality of the content and biologic activity of the herbal remedies on the market. One cannot assume that the black cohosh purchased under one label is the same offered at the drugstore under another label. Thus, in 1972, the OTC Review at the FDA began the evaluation of all ingredients used in OTC products with the intent of requiring a higher standard in the processing of OTC herbal therapies. Yet products labeled "natural" do not automatically mean "safe." And then there is the issue of adverse drug reactions that have been associated with herbal remedies and the interaction of prescription drugs. Saint-John's-wort, a popular OTC herbal medicine used by many in the United States for depression, has been shown to decrease the metabolism of a number of drugs. Some herb products taken for their diuretic property interact with lithium given for bipolar depression. The bottom line is that prescribing clinicians must ask clients, "What over-the-counter supplements are you taking?" before prescribing a new medication. And likewise, clients taking prescribed therapies need to inform their health care providers before adding a new supplement. Pharmacists can also be a helpful resource regarding supplements. The options for herbal therapies are discussed at length in chapter 5.

PERSONAL EMPOWERMENT STRATEGIES

Although you may note some overlap in the following section on emotional well-being and strategies for enhancement, I could not conclude this chapter without a deeper journey into these specific *personal empowerment strategies.* Let's begin with *spirituality.* My definition of spirituality is a "personal relationship" between a person and her God or higher power. Traditional religions possess doctrine, traditions, rituals, and practices of worship. Spirituality from my perspective is that inner foundation of faith, hope, and trust that is demonstrated through prayer, meditation, solitude, gratitude, simplicity, harmony, and personal growth. The late twentieth century brought the advent of the New Age movement, a practice regarding spirituality as an active and vital connection to a force/power/energy, spirit, or deep sense of self. Conduct a word search on the Internet for "spirituality," and you'll find a plethora of links to Christian spirituality, holistic spirituality, Jewish spirituality, Native American spirituality, Catholic spirituality, New Age spirituality and so on. The point is that personal empowerment offers one an opportunity to transcend daily living with faith, hope, and prayer for a journey into inner growth of the spirit. What is your spiritual life holding for you today? What beliefs or practices bring you harmony of mind, body, and spirit? This menopause transition for some opens a new path to inner growth and speculation. I have a suggestion for those wanting to delve deeper into spirituality: go to your favorite bookstore with at least two hours at your disposal. Visit the New Age, spiritual, or religion section and peruse. Pick up at least three books that strike your fancy and skim the tables of contents. What interests you?

For a profound experience, visit a sacred place—a church, a cathedral, a holy place, or even a location like Sedona, Arizona. While visiting Italy on our honeymoon several years ago, my poor husband, Brad, was drug into just about every church in every town we explored. One memorable afternoon was at the Sacro Monte of Varallo. Basilicas and chapels created by the Milanese Franciscan friar Father Bernardino Caimi in the fifteenth century are nestled up in the mountains. A "miniature Holy Land" with 43 chapels, each depicting a story from Adam and Eve to the Holy Sepulchre where Jesus lay after his death, are represented in this sacred city. But if a trip to Italy is not on the agenda, look for a retreat center or quiet place to rest your spirit undisturbed. Several weeks ago, a writer's block had cast a spell over my creative forces. A colleague, a client, and a newspaper story told of a retreat center in the woods of western North Carolina. It was not a coincidence that three separate forces invited me to the "Well of Mercy." Many thanks to the Sisters of Mercy for their vision in creating this quiet sanctuary and the respectful hospitality they provide to their guests. Twenty-four hours of rest and renewal was just what I needed. Find a sacred intersection in your daily round for renewal. *Spirit* may just find you on an early morning walk; while folding clothes, in a yoga class, or planning a delicious meal for two; or on a quiet evening wrapped in a blanket before a roaring fire.

Anaïs Nin remarked, "Each friend represents a world in us, a world possibly not born until they arrive, and it is only by this meeting that a new world is born." How many *friends* can you call a "true friend," one who supports you through emotional difficulties and physical challenges and who empathizes with your situation without letting you rest too long on your rear end? A 2006 study cites that the number and quality of friendships for the average American has declined since 1985.[9] Can it be true that 25 percent of Americans have no close confidants and that the average number of confidants per person has dropped to two? Is that due to busy lives, complacency, or self-involvement? Many women share their sadness that a geographic move left them with long-distance friendships but not a local kindred spirit to share time with. The colorful threads weaving a tapestry of friendship are trust, honesty, mutual understanding, affection, and loyalty. Those intimate chats, confessions, and long night ministries provided by a friend do indeed warm the heart. Being fortunate to have a friend requires that you treat them with love and respect and nurture the unconditional love they shower on you. What have you done lately to nurture a special one in your life? Have you told your confidant that you love and honor the relationship in words and actions? The following are a few examples of treasuring them beyond words: send special cards for no reason at all, bring back a present when you take a trip, celebrate life changes together (those special birthdays at ages 40, 50, 60, and 70 because this generation can live that long), take trips to the beach, build annual traditions, call and send notes during difficult times, take spa trips to rejuvenate, deliver care baskets when they are sick, and be there when a loved one passes away. The blessing of friends—having one and being one—calls on the essence within to rise up and be present even when it is inconvenient. My dear Lorie has taught me much about the heart of a friend. She was there living across the street as we raised our children, seeking advice and sharing the challenges. She kept my spirit balanced through a painful divorce. And she stood beside me when I said, "I do!" to Brad. These days we talk, share little joys as perimenopausal women, compliment each other on the fabulous job of raising these 20-year-olds, and plan that next getaway together. Friendship—yes, another force of personal empowerment.

I believe the importance of friendship will take baby boomer women into a new lifestyle option your mother never considered: communal living. Boomer women are accustomed to controlling their own lives, business, and finances. They lived together in dorms, and sororities. They shared apartments after college. Many traveled together and found great comfort in the arms of friendship through difficult life passages such as divorce or loss of a child. And many of this population will outlive their partners by at least seven years and expect to be widows; aging with friends may just be the answer. My dear friends and I tease often during our girls' weekends that we will indeed live together, pooling our resources, continuing to share life's challenges, and hiring a cabana boy to push our wheelchairs onto the dock and load us into the boat for those sunsets of our golden years.

I cannot present the next section without a thank-you to Sarah Ban Breathnach. Her book *Simple Abundance: A Daybook of Comfort and Joy* has been a dear companion of mine for years. For many women, this book opened the world of authenticity through daily *affirmations*. Her six practical, creative, and spiritual principles are gratitude, simplicity, order, harmony, beauty, and joy. What a treasure this book has been for many women struggling with their identity. The affirmations embedded in her message soothe the spirit.

Affirmations are the self-talk and inner dialogue to affirm the subconscious through our words and thoughts. The mind is in constant motion. It explores one's environment and tries to "read the room." What if the room is filled with negative messages? What if the view from the mind's window is dark and fear filled, leading to avoidance? Positive affirmations can wash away the negative tapes and messages you carry in your mind. When spoken too frequently, injunctions such as "Menopause is a horrific time of life" or "How will I ever get past these hot flashes and be me again?" can taint the mind and limit possibilities. "I am able to breathe through this hot flash, knowing it is a temporary condition"—doesn't that sound positive? "I am a resilient, centered woman able to challenge every curve in the road of my menopause journey"—again, a positive frame of reference. Positive affirmations are short positive statements targeted to challenge negative beliefs or a set of assumptions. Using affirmations to reprogram thought patterns changes the way you think and feel about issues by replacing the dysfunctional or toxic beliefs. A focus of my work with women entering menopause is to reflect on their thinking and beliefs regarding menopause. Challenging the inner voice with positive daily affirmations moves many past the gridlock of negativity.

Bookstores abound with affirmation books; Amazon listed more than 1,700 at the time of this writing. I have several favorites I want to share. *Time for Joy Daily Journal: A Pocket Book of Affirmations* by Ruth Fishel and *Meditations for Women Who Do Too Much* by Anne Wilson are two worth checking out. My suggestion to clients is to find a book that speaks to you, purchase it, and read it three times a day to imprint the positive message. Write it down in your journal and use sticky notes on your mirror, in the car, on your desk, and in your day planner to hasten the process. After three weeks of daily readings and thought, the mind is washed of its negative debris, and positive uplifting beliefs become natural. You creative spirits may want to make your own affirmations. Begin your phrase in first person, using the present tense: "I am". The remaining text highlights your new belief: "I am living life beautifully as a menopausal woman."

The next personal empowerment strategy may bump up against a message from a parent or teacher from your past: *daydreaming*. I believe that daydreaming is another manifestation of a healthy mind. Sometimes mental imagery can help a client gain insight into her own mental state. For the voyager in the menopause passage, let your mind wander, let imagination flourish, and let creativity become your muse. Historically, daydreaming has had a bad rap. It has been associated with laziness. How many times did an adult tell you to get your head out of the clouds, focus on the task at hand, and stop that lazy behavior? Some studies suggest that those with a high aptitude for daydreaming have more empathy. It might be said that a daydream is an eyes-wide-open, visual fantasy. To connect with your daytime fantasy, suspend conscious thought and reality, keep your eyes open, sit and relax, open your mind, and suspend time for 15 minutes. Deliberately focus on the scene in your mind's eye—possibly a future experience, a pleasant setting, or the seasoned woman you remain at age 80. Make the scene as realistic and detailed as possible, coloring the scene with your senses until it triggers an emotional response. The emotional response could be joy, contentment, relief of today's worries, and serenity. Launching these moments of fantasy mobilizes the creative and relaxed you—a much-needed state of being in this busy world.

Did you ever consider movie watching as empowering? Sara Ban Breathnach suggested just such an exceptional idea in her book for the August 26 meditation. Surrender your critical parent voice and consider this: you slip into the dark of the theater, box of popcorn in hand, a silent void of responsibility, two hours of pure delight, and entertainment at its height. This entertainment can be from any genre, be it mystery, drama, action, comedy, or family viewing. The point is to relax and enjoy while the possibility of discerning insight from the power of celluloid sweeps through. Some films are uplifting, encourage the human spirit, and send a potent message to the viewer.

Sometime this week, journey to the video store with paper and pen in hand. Glide through the aisle jotting down movies of interest—those you have never seen before or the movie that spoke to you in a previous life that you want to revisit in the present-day you. Then within the next month, I suggest you take a day off for your own date with movie watching. Take your list, select a few for the day, pop the corn, and sit back and *enjoy*.

The final strategy to enliven your spirit comes in dualistic presentation. Learn to say "no" and learn to play hooky. How can these two be related? When was the last time you tried to play hooky? If never, you do not know of the dilemma I speak of. Playing hooky requires you to say "no." "No, I cannot be at the meeting." "No, I cannot pick up your laundry this morning." "No, the project will have to find another chairperson." Mastery in the art of saying "no" takes a lifetime to perfect. I began my pursuit of its art many years ago.

My husband and children might tell you, "She has not arrived yet." The early years of raising children, being an attentive wife, growing a successful private practice, and being involved in the nursing community and director of the social calendar escalated the necessity for "no" responses. The superwoman syndrome had me by the throat until "no" became my traveling companion. Today I invite each of you to assess your ability to utter this brief but potent phrase. How many times over the past month did you accept a social request and then wish you had said, "Thank you, but we are unable to join you"? Ponder the upcoming week's agenda and write it down. Then commit to saying "yes" to only the essentials to make the week's agenda viable and "no" to the other options you might be seduced to accept. This week you are that seasoned woman in her second adulthood, which no longer needs to please or perform for authority figures. You are strong in your own convictions of authenticity and balance.

Now for playing hooky. As a nurse practitioner, I subscribe to "mental health days" and "playing hooky." Let's differentiate between the two. Mental health days are when you are too weary to take another step toward responsibility. On such days, you call in to the office, tell the family you are "off the clock," and do just about nothing except rest and refuel. You likely either have experienced the need for a mental health day or have taken one. But what about playing hooky? When did you last write "playing hooky" on your day planner and center the day around *play*? "Play" means taking a full eight-hour span of time for fun—and on a workday, too. Play is necessary for your good health—emotional, physical, and sexual. Be self-indulgent and tap into idleness. Make an appointment at the local day spa for a pedicure, facial, and body soak. Take yourself to lunch or go to a movie that you might not otherwise attend. Play a round of golf all by yourself. Or, if play means inviting that special person to join you, then include him or her in your play. Maybe a nap and a good book are more your style of play. The activity you choose is less important than the central theme of "me time."

Chapter Eight

SEXUAL REVITALIZATION

And the day came when the risk to remain tight in a bud was more painful than the risk it took to blossom.

—Anaïs Nin

Lexie wanted more than the lukewarm sexual relationship she had for 14 years with Ben. In that first session, she admitted in a shy manner that she had experienced only one orgasm, and that was the previous summer after feeling really close and excited by Ben. She wondered if it was too late to even try for orgasms. Yet for me, the major question was not whether she could have an orgasm but what was getting in the way of her sexual spirit?

> We have been married 14 years and dated five years before marriage. Ben and I decided to wait for intercourse. But we did pretty much everything else. It was fun. I couldn't wait to see him and explore the new sexual connection. It was so *hot*, she said. Then we got married and pretty much as soon as I said "I do" the sexual excitement went away. I will take responsibility for part of the loss of excitement. But, Ben is just so "goal oriented" and the goal has been his pleasure not pleasing me. My part of the problem is I don't know what I need to get more excited and have an orgasm. Now that I am starting to have hot flashes I also find the sensations 'down there' are not as strong. Do you think you can help us?

Women often enter therapy wondering if they are so unusual or so "messed up" that there is no hope. I applaud Lexie and women like her for stretching beyond her comfort zone and seeking the sometimes hidden treasure of sexual pleasure. Lexie's story is compounded by the onset of perimenopausal symptoms—it isn't impossible to tap into that dormant sexual "well of pleasure" during the menopause transition. It does require courage to explore barriers to pleasure those unresolved relationship issues or perhaps external factors such as work commitments or time demands and then tap into determination and patience. Her profile is not entirely unique. Other stories involve the woman who has been orgasmic and enjoyed a full range of sexual activities with her partner; however, now the sensations are dull, energy is less because of lack of sleep, and her body image is more negative from the weight gain. This woman is a perfect candidate for "sexual revitalization," a term first seen in print related to the sexual teachings of the Jade Dragon and the Taoist methods of male sexual revitalization.[1] Gail Sheehy was the next author utilizing the term to describe the women interviewed for her book *Sex and the Seasoned Woman: Pursuing the Passionate Life.*[2] Many of the women either in long-term marriages or single again described a desire to reignite their sexuality in spite of symptoms related to menopause; they were just not willing to give up the joys of sexuality. For some long-married couples, a new spark develops with the "resurgence of romantic love and sexual intimacy once the children leave," remarks Sheehy.[3]

Yet, regardless of the length of time in the relationship or a woman's rich development of her sexuality, menopause is a perfect opportunity to launch a new sexual identity or enhance the sexual spirit.

In the rhythm of life, a couple falls into and out of love many times in the course of a long-term marriage. Fluctuations could be from internal or external forces, such as distractions from work, demands of child rearing, and a perceived lack of time to nurture the relationship. I am a firm believer that those who once loved passionately can indeed revive the passion when incidents of life rob them of their sexual zest. Keeping sex a satisfying element in a relationship requires communication of one's needs and time to nurture the sexual spirit.

Judith Wallerstein, one of America's leading experts on marriage and author of the book *The Good Marriage: How and Why Love Lasts*, focused her research on 50 married couples who considered themselves happily married. "A rich rewarding and stable sex life is not just a fringe benefit. It is the central task of marriage," she states. Pertaining to long-term married couples, she believes that "a revitalization of sex life is what refuels the marriage of those who approach midlife."[4]

Steve Slon, editor in chief of *AARP Magazine* states, "Baby Boomers believe that they invented sex, and they still think so." Although boomers may not have invented sex, they expanded the meaning and the menu. In fact, a recent study revealed that the boomer generation really is different from generations past both in behaviors and in overall attitude. Steve Slon remarked in a magazine story, "A strong majority [of boomers] say sex is a critical ingredient in their lifestyle. Sixty some percent of them say they are having sex once a week. And two-thirds of midlife couples say they are satisfied with their midlife sex lives."[5] This is certainly a different picture than the intimacy and sex lives of midlife adults in the Veteran generation. Think back to the television programs of the 1950s with twin beds in the bedrooms of the *Leave It to Beaver* and *I Love Lucy* programs. You didn't see Ward Cleaver giving June a passionate embrace or steeling off for a little sexual play. Compare those sitcoms with today's programs, such as *Sex in the City*, *Grey's Anatomy*, and *The View*, as well as the reality shows that invade the homes of families every night.

In 1999, American Association of Retired Persons (AARP) boldly conducted a landmark survey of adults age 45 and older, "Sexuality at Midlife and Beyond." Their objective was to understand the role sex plays in quality for life of midlife and older adults. The results were published in *Modern Maturity* magazine and on the AARP Web site. The AARP commissioned the research group again in 2004 to repeat the 1999 sexuality study and add a new section in an attempt to understand the differences in sexual attitudes and behaviors of racial/ethnic groups: whites, African Americans, Hispanics, and Asians. Eighty-six percent of the surveys were returned with 1,682 respondents in the study. The mean was 61 years of age. Two-thirds of the persons reported that they were married, one-fourth were divorced or widowed, and 4 percent of males and 1 percent of females reported same-sex partners.[6]

Sexual attitudes from the 2004 survey report sexuality remains an essential element in the lives of U.S. adults age 45 and older. More than one-half reported sexual activity as a critical part of a good relationship and that a satisfying sexual relationship is an important factor in quality of life. Those with a regular sex partner noted a better chance of being sexually satisfied than nonpartnered respondents. Regarding health issues, the majority believe that health affects sexual satisfaction. And the number of adults seeking treatment for a sexual functioning problem is growing, with an increase in the use of medicines, hormones, or other treatments to improve their sexual lives. Fifteen percent of women take hormones within the 50–59 age-group. The 2004 survey notes an increase use of medications for high blood pressure and elevated cholesterol. These are the most common medical conditions respondents have been diagnosed with. In general, women are twice more likely to experience depression than men. Thirty-one percent of men reported impotence, while 5 percent reported that prescription medications were taken to improve sexual functioning.[7]

It is heartening to see an increase of attention to the sexual attitudes and behaviors of midlife adults. The AARP has taken the lead where our conservative government groups continue to sit back and watch sexual vitality for our youth and the aging change the face of the nation. What will the next 5 to

10 years uncover for midlife Americans? A well-used statistic is that "in the United States, 6,000 women a day enter menopause." Can growth of such a substantial group and their needs continue to be downplayed?

BABY BOOMERS AS SEX EDUCATORS

Boomers were the first generation to receive sex education in the public school classroom. Yet peer groups probably had a stronger influence on sexual behaviors and early exploration of this population. Boomer parents often abdicated their role as sex educator because of their own parents' ignorance as role models and the fear that they did not have the facts or skill to teach this controversial subject. Who taught the Veteran generation parents, the parents of boomers, their sexual lessons?

I firmly believe that parents should be the primary sex educator of children to teach sexual health and responsible sexual behavior. If parents do not accept the responsibility and begin early, the peer group or an individual's faltering exploration will prevail. Where did your sex education come from? Did your parents give you a book to read? Some menopausal women state that the "sex talk" was given once but that questions were not invited. Those were the lucky ones. In my years as a sex therapist and presenter on this subject, more often I heard the tales of "no sex story" and "no sex book." Instead, baby boomers went limping into the arena of sexuality guided by their own ignorance or peer group teachings. In 1995, as a new parent of a curious eight-year-old boy, I found his questions concerning sex a challenge even for this sex therapist. Wanting to give appropriate answers, I ran, not walked, to the bookstore. Absent were books for the parents of latency children, those children ages 8 to 12. *When Benjamin Wants to Know: Family Conversations about the Facts of Life* became my rendering for parents like me who wanted to tackle this sex educator role for 8- to 12-year-olds.[8] Publishing companies did not believe a market existed for the subject. Had they been in the bookstores lately? Were they parents of a curious boy like Ben?

Benjamin's book is told in first person; it really is his story, and Ben did all the initial drawings for the manuscript. The book is a bold testament for other parents wanting to educate sexually inquisitive youth. We wrote the book for parents to read to children or to give that probing child so that he or she could read a specific chapter, then parents could answer provoking questions. Morning conversations while dressing for work and school seemed to be just the right time for Ben's questions, or in the car on the way to school—another perfect time to unsettle a parent.

The other platform for my message became opportunities for public speaking. Various parent groups, PTA meetings, day care settings, nursing groups, and other health care professional groups heard and responded to "Speaking of Sex: How to Be an 'Askable' Parent." Never did a presentation conclude before five or six parents came up to share their stories. By far, the common thread was that many received no information from their parents. Now to complete the companion book for girls, *When Jessica Wants to Know: Family Conversations about the Facts of Life.* I am a believer that if this generation responds to the challenge and becomes "askable" parents—those who look for "teachable moments"—their children will possess strong sexual identities free from the sexual ignorance we struggled through.

Former U.S. Surgeon General David Satcher convened leaders of major constituency organizations with interests in sexual health to participate in a consensus process on sexual health in 2004 as a follow-up to his bold 2001 report, "The Surgeon General's Call to Action to Promote Sexual Health and Responsible Sexual Behavior." In May 2006, the Interim Report of the National Consensus Process on Sexual Health and Responsible Sexual Behaviors was released. Although significant areas of agreement were reached on key issues, areas of continued disagreement persist, such as sexual abstinence, responsible sexual behavior, and sexual orientation. I was pleased to see examples of consensus regarding core elements of sexuality education as well as a common vision of what constitutes sexual health. Parents are acknowledged as critical providers of sexual education. The interim report includes components of sound education to help guide parents from modeling to practices.[9] I applaud the work of the group and their commitment to continue the consensus process toward the goal of improving sexual health in America. This is just another legacy that today's menopausal women and their partners leave to the following generations beyond breaking through glass ceilings, insisting on a voice for their health care choices, and reinventing the golden years beyond retirement.

SEXUAL MYTHS

Sex stops at age 50. Can it be that even in the twenty-first century we cling to some old, crippling myths regarding sex and the midlife couple? Admittedly, low sexual desire is cited by many clinicians as the top sexual complaint in marriages. Often men protest that sex is not frequent enough for their liking. Although some women share this concern, far more women utter the need for "quality in their lovemaking." The inhibiting factors of too little time and too little energy often leave couples celibate in their later years. Therapists who encourage couples to vent their sexual needs in a caring fashion while a partner actively listens can unlock even the rustiest lock on sexual satisfaction.[10]

I remember years ago watching Lonnie Barbach's video *Sex after 50*. The "man on the street" was queried about midage adults and sexuality; even this population of mature persons said, "Sex stops at 50 or at least by age 58." Lonnie's comment to these statements was that "our culture denies seniors their sexuality." The video was made in 1991. Now, I ask you, have things really changed? The 2004 AARP sexuality survey reported that of their 1,682 respondents, 6 out of 10 agree that sexual activity is a critical part of a good relationship, and about half agree that sexual activity is important to their overall quality of life. Finally, the vast majority disagree that sex is only for the younger people.[11]

Lonnie breaks through the myth that sex stops at age 50. It is a great video, one I have sent home for many couples to review. My favorite recipient was an 80-year-old gentleman who had lost his wife to cancer. He was referred to me by a colleague. At a college reunion on the East Coast, he renewed a relationship with a woman he had known decades before. Her husband was also deceased for many years. In their reacquaintance, they rediscovered love. This captivating gentleman wanted to recharge his sexual battery and determine the best manner to broach the subject with his lady. A few therapy sessions, sharing Lonnie's video, and another trip to visit his lady found them both eager to renew passion and explore the wonders of sexual revitalization. I heard from my colleague that his lady became his wife, they enjoyed their love for only a short year, and the remarkable gentleman died. I did receive a Christmas card from "his lady"; she thanked me for the year of love and passion. So no, sex does not end at age 50.

Sex must always be spontaneous. This is an outrageous myth at any age. For the midlife woman, a natural happening is very possible but not on every occasion. Many of the women I work with are exploring methods of reigniting their sexual flame when the hormonal challenges of hot flashes or an elusive state of desire are ever present. They often need to take time to coordinate the sexual mind-set with the body's pleasure zones, and that is not a spontaneous process.

Another factor to consider regarding this myth is that for today's fast-paced world, planning and scheduling are the only sure ways to protect your priorities. Making sexual connection a priority, not just a happenstance, increases overall satisfaction in a relationship. Date nights are popular with couples, but planning very brief sexual encounters and leisurely interludes keeps sex alive. One-third of midlife adults in the 2004 AARP survey stated that they have sexual intercourse regularly (once a week or more often). More than one-half engage in sexual touching or caressing, and around two-thirds kiss or hug their partner on a regular basis. Oral sex and self-stimulation are not as prevalent as the other sexual activities.[12] So even in the golden years, time is indeed carved out for touch, loving caress, and intercourse.

Sex always takes a certain amount of time to be successful. Not one of the many hundreds of men I have worked with in the over 20 years of sex therapy has ever shown me this rule in the "Guide to Being a Great Lover Handbook." I am being sarcastic about the handbook, yet I have wondered for as many years where boys learn to be sexual partners. Or should I say learn to be attentive partners. I pose this question for many a couple when they enter therapy to resolve issues of low desire or performance anxiety. Women share the hope that their first sexual experience is with a partner who knows just how to pleasure her. Where do they think this young man got his preparation to be a "lover" much less a great one? If parents are the primary sex educators for children, how many of you parents shared the lesson of "great lover" with either your daughter or son? So who did? The peer group again rises to the occasion. And then there is old-fashioned "on the job training" subtitled "learning loving together."

A certain amount of time for sex is just ridiculous as a rule for lovemaking. Take whatever amount of time feels good. There is absolutely nothing wrong with "the quickie"; each style of lovemaking has its own pleasant amount of time equated to it. My recommendation to couples in all age-groups is to explore the many styles of lovemaking and have variety as your benchmark. Later in this chapter when we get to "strategies" to revitalize the sexual spirit, I share styles of lovemaking that I developed for the Sexplore Weekend Retreats I provide for couples.

This last myth is my favorite to debunk. *Sex must always end in orgasm.* The believer of this myth is often not a woman. Chasing orgasms versus focusing time and attention to "building mutual pleasure" is a crippling sexual belief. Orgasms are delightful. They are, however, only one component in a couple's "sexual menu." A sexual menu includes appetizers, side dishes, and the main course. Orgasms reside in the main course. Imagine all the appetizers a couple can invent to awaken passion, desire, and dismiss boredom. Sexual menus are discussed later in this chapter. It has been an "in-session" exercise for many couples I work with. And when they commit to exploring their present menu and enhancing it with variety and playfulness, boredom no longer resides in the bedroom.

How comfortable are midlife adults in asking a partner to try a sex-related activity? The 2004 AARP survey reports that one-half of respondents would either try an activity or ask their partner to try. The most frequently mentioned sex activity was watching adult films with a partner, followed by using sex toys and engaging in erotic notes or e-mails. Two changes from the 1999 survey I found interesting were an increase in the proportion of men and women engaging in self-stimulation, and more males report engaging in oral sex now compared to 1999.[13]

SEXUALITY CHANGES IN MIDLIFE

Sexuality changes as we age, relationships evolve, and a person's well-being grows or declines. This is all normal. If a woman enjoyed sex before menopause, she more than likely will enjoy sexuality after the transition. The sexually mature woman is more experienced and knows what to ask for and how to tap into her senses to ignite passion and move to desire. Postmenopausal women who did not enjoy their sexual connection before may find a more pronounced decrease in their desire for sexual activity. The key for the menopausal woman is to acknowledge that your body is or has changed, discuss changes with your partner, and realize that you may now require more stimulation and time to achieve the pleasurable sensations of yesteryear. Setting up realistic expectations for your sexual relationship with your partner is vital. When a woman is less available now than before, her partner might misread this as "she is not attracted to me anymore" when in fact the attraction is still there but her ability to arouse her mind and body more difficult. The majority of women find they have to be more intentional in igniting the mind with the body. They need more time to "warm up" to sex and transition from businesswoman, homemaker, or grandmother into sexual diva. The classic multitasking world you live in has to be downshifted to allow for sex. For some, another hurdle is the faulty thinking one has toward oneself as a vibrant available partner or faulty thinking about the partner. And many men also need more time to get a firm erection, and visual stimulation alone may not be as reliable an igniter. Believing that spontaneous desire will move you to act sexually in midlife as you did in at age 20 is a sure recipe for disappointment. A reasonable framework for sexual expectations is that sometimes sex will be great, sometimes sex will be good, and sometimes sex will be less than desirable.

Lorie, a 58-year-old woman, entered therapy some three years after her last period. "I find my lubrication has changed, so now sexual intercourse is a little painful. But my biggest fear is my once-excited response to my man's touch and his attention has decreased. I do not want to give up sex. I have always enjoyed it—well, after the kids got a little older and were less demanding. Matt and I want to travel. We enjoy our alone time, and I 'want' him as much now as before. What are my options?"

Lorie and women like her are ever present in a health care provider's office. They are the brave souls who will not fall prey to old stereotypes that midlife women are unattractive or uninterested in sex. Menopause does not signal the end of sexual pleasure. Lorie added a vaginal moisturizer, Liquibeads by K-Y. These long-lasting beads restore vaginal moisture lasting up to four days. She augmented this strategy with Astroglide, a personal lubricant applied to her genitals during intercourse to decrease further painful friction. Matt and Lorie talked more about their expectations for this sexual passage. "How frequently do we want to have intercourse? What other ways of being affectionate and loving can we add to our sexual menu?" And they realized that spending more time sexually stimulating each other and the use of a small vibrator did wonders to enhance their already strong sexual connection. "I didn't realize how simply adding a sense of 'playfulness' to our sexual connection could bring back such excitement," Lorie commented in her last session.

To simplify a complex process that was discussed in great detail in chapter 2, let's take a snapshot of this normal process of aging for women that is experienced by most at about age 52. Prior to the end of menses, many women notice a cascade of body changes, from irregular menstrual cycles, hot flashes, and a decrease in vaginal lubrication to that dreaded sleep cycle disruption. Chronic sleep disturbance establishes negative changes in mood and overall well-being. The ovaries stop releasing eggs, and menstrual periods stop. Changes in hormone activity set the stage for all these bodily experiences. The sex hormones estrogen, progesterone, testosterone, and prolactin also decrease around menopause. As hormone levels fall, changes occur throughout the reproductive system. The vagina shortens, secretions decrease, and the vaginal walls become thin and less elastic, sometimes creating pain with intercourse (dyspareunia). And the external genital tissue of the labia loses shape and elasticity. These last few symptoms are more common in the first few years of postmenopause.

Changes within the urinary system can also occur as the vagina; the uterus and urinary bladder lose muscle tone and can be displaced in the body. These changes can set into motion urine leakage or stress incontinence when a woman sneezes, laughs hard, runs, or exercises. The good news is that most of these conditions can be treated.

Loss of muscle tone, the sagging of breast tissue, loss of skin elasticity, and an increased risk for osteoporosis further complicate body changes for women in response to loss of hormone function. Even with the many changes possible during transition into menopause, the symptoms vary in severity. Only about 20 to 30 percent of all women have symptoms severe enough to seek medical or hormone treatment.

Some of the Sexual Changes Are the Following
- Less natural lubrication produced during sex
- Vaginal walls get thinner and may make intercourse uncomfortable
- Slower sexual arousal
- Intensity of orgasms may be reduced
- Skin sensitivity may be increased or decrease

Although a common belief is that hormone changes during the menopause transition are the culprit for sexual desire to decline, as a sex therapist I believe it is a more complicated picture. The combination of hormonal, health, and social changes associated with aging and the emotional effects of the transition can work together to dampen desire. However, just as the hormonal process for women is changing, men are also experiencing a decline in testosterone and find that they too need additional stimulation to tap into those higher levels of arousal. Thus couples can enrich the experience for both by slowing down, stimulating not only the body but also the relationship with "out-of-the-bedroom connections."

Paula Doress-Worters, author of *The New Ourselves, Growing Older*, states that "there is no reason to think that women in midlife should necessarily have problems with sexuality. Although menopause does bring physiologic changes that may slow down response time 70%–80% of women do not experience a reduction in sexual activity or satisfaction."[14] In fact, some women have a reawakening of sexuality, no longer concerned about getting pregnant; able to take more time for lovemaking, they know what they are doing, and adult children require less time and attention.

SEXUAL DYSFUNCTION IN THE MENOPAUSE YEARS

Women often remain silent for months or years before voicing a concern regarding their sexual health. A *sexual dysfunction* is a persistent or recurrent disturbance in the process of the sexual response cycle or pain associated with sexual intercourse causing an individual marked distress or interpersonal difficulty. The *Diagnostic and Statistical Manual of Mental Disorders* (*DSM-IV*) has long been the bible for mental health professionals. Participants at the International Consultation on Sexual Medicine held in Paris in June 2003 challenged many of the previously held beliefs regarding women's sexual response. The defining elements of sexual dysfunction within *DSM-IV* are on the absence of sexual fantasy and genital swelling and lubrication. In other words, the *DSM-IV* and female sexual dysfunction are focused on the genitals. These are poor indicators for a woman's subjective sexual arousal and pleasure. The proposed new descriptions for categories of sexual disorders can be found in the book *The Science of Orgasm* by Beverly Whipple.[15]

Probably the largest challenge in a reliable diagnosis for female sexual dysfunction relates to a woman's experience of desire. Dr. Rosemary Basson, one of the leading researchers in this area, believes that desire does not follow a linear progression as first described by Masters and Johnson, that a woman's sexual response is more circular with overlapping phases, and that desire is triggered *after* moderate levels of arousal, not at the onset of sexual activity.[16] Health care providers working with women's sexual health have one major responsibility before labeling her lack of desire or difficulty with arousal as "the issue": providers must first evaluate her physical, emotional, and relationship well-being to assess dysfunction. Far too often, the sexual difficulty is not lifelong; it is often situational or from an ongoing loss of connection in the relationship or in midlife from hormonal changes.

A study from the National Health and Social Life Survey indicates that nearly one-half of U.S. women (and midlife is no exception) report one or more difficulties with their sexual health.[17] These include *hypoactive sexual desire disorders, sexual arousal disorders, orgasmic disorders,* and *sexual pain disorders.* Why does it take so long for a woman to voice her concerns? A 1999 survey showed that 71 percent of patients believed their physician would dismiss sexual concerns, 68 percent believed their physician would be embarrassed by a discussion of sexual problems, and 76 percent did not think treatments were available to help with sexual concerns.[18] So we in the health care arena have dropped the ball by not asking the sexual questions during annual physical exams or other points of care. Medical and nursing schools need to desensitize students to sexual issues so that providers can ask these pertinent questions without embarrassment. Patients have a right to be asked about all facets of their health by their provider, and patients need to know that even if a health care provider does not address your sexual concern, you can. We often call these *doorknob confessions,* or the last few concerns a patient utters before exiting the treatment room. More recently, in seminars I conduct to desensitize clinicians to sexual topics, I encourage nurses and physicians to schedule an additional session within a few days to deal with the concerns dropped at the doorknob. Delaying the appointment only silences that fearful voice, whether the voice is the provider or the patient.

Female Sexual Dysfunctions Include the Following

- Hypoactive sexual desire disorders
- Sexual arousal disorders
- Orgasmic disorders
- Sexual pain disorders

Hypoactive Sexual Desire Disorder

Decline in hormone levels varies from woman to woman, and although the decline can produce a change in sexual function, many factors can be responsible for the loss of sexual satisfaction. These include relationship concerns, psychological issues, biologic factors, health concerns, absence of a partner, and, a major contributing factor, a woman's perception of her body. It is fairly common to have sexual dysfunction issues in more than one category. Treatments can in fact overlap and help with more than one problem.

There is no "normal" level of sexual response—it is different in every woman and in each sexual encounter. Normal sexual response is a personal critique based on a woman's motivation and interest, her sexual arousability, and her response to stimulus. What may feel normal or satisfying to you at one stage of your life changes at another stage or age. At the core of sexuality for women is a need for closeness and intimacy.

Utilizing Dr. Basson's model for "female sexual response," a woman does not begin the process with sexual desire; she is more sexually neutral. As her motivation for sex or her reason to initiate or agree to sex becomes positive, she moves to a state of willingness to receive and respond to sexual stimulation. This state of subjective arousal and continued stimulation increases her sense of excitement and pleasure, "triggering" sexual desire. The desire that was absent at the onset of the sexual experience can now ignite further sexual satisfaction, with or without orgasm, as long as she remains focused and receives sufficient stimulation for orgasm.[19] This is a very different process than the 1966 research by Masters and Johnson. I spend a great deal of time educating woman about the changes in this model to assist their new understanding regarding their interest, motivation, willingness to respond, level of stimulus needed for heightened levels of arousal, the onset of desire, and ultimately their need to remain focused on pleasure and not let "time" disrupt the process.

If you notice a change in sexual desire or sexual satisfaction, take a look at what is and what is not working with your body and your life. Ask a few pertinent questions:

- Am I stressed more than usual?
- Is there a physical reason for the loss of desire?
- Am I taking any medications that could dampen my desire?
- Is my body image interfering with desire?
- Do I get aroused thinking about sex? Do I stop the arousal in any way?
- Do I have an honest, caring, respectful connection with my partner?
- Am I able to identify my own sexual needs and communicate them to my partner?
- Do we make our sexual connection a priority and take the time we need?
- Are we consistently nurturing our relationship outside the bedroom?
- Are there sexual issues from the past that get in the way of today's pleasure?

A *diagnosis of hypoactive sexual desire* is made when there is a persistent and recurrent absence of sexual fantasy, diminished feelings of sexual interest, or lack of responsive desire for sexual activity causing personal distress. A population study of adults 18 to 59 years of age by Laumann, author of *Sex in America,* revealed that sexual dysfunction is more prevalent for women (43%) than men (31%).[20] A 2004 study by Plaut reports an increase in sexual dysfunction for women after menopause to 45 percent.[21] As I mentioned earlier, many factors can lower libido, such as adrenal fatigue, conflictual relationships, stress, health concerns, and a complex lifestyle. Adequate amounts of testosterone and estrogen (estradiol) are vitally important in promoting healthy libido. If you suffer from low desire, examining your free testosterone by saliva testing or blood levels to determine your normal level is helpful. Testosterone is in a group of sex hormones known as androgens. Another androgen dehydroepiandrosterone (DHEA), important in the process of desire, is discussed later in this section. In fact, the body possesses several avenues to produce testosterone. Two primary manufacturers are the adrenal glands and the ovaries. Women suffering from androgen insufficiency can find themselves in a struggle for sexual energy; thus, DHEA, even though its use is controversial at this time, may be another option for that lagging desire. Dr. Susan Rako, a psychiatrist and the author of *The Hormone of Desire: The Truth about Sexuality, Menopause and Testosterone,* believes that testosterone therapy is a major breakthrough for midlife women and can prevent much unnecessary anguish.[22] Although androgen therapy remains controversial, anecdotal notes from clinicians and women, along with several small studies, suggest that individualized doses added to estrogen therapy can boost both testosterone and energy.

Estradiol, the smallest in the estrogen hormone group but by far the most active, is a by-product of testosterone. When estrogen levels drop, testosterone takes another hit on its production process. There is a 50 percent fall in a woman's testosterone by ages 20 to 45. Then, by the end of menopause, testosterone is down by 90 percent.[23] What can you do to promote testosterone production in your body during this phase of depletion? First, evaluate your baseline level of circulating testosterone. Testosterone products available on the market may be an option; they are used "off label," meaning that testosterone therapy for women is not approved for women by the Food and Drug Administration (FDA) For many years, men were given this option for low testosterone levels, yet it is controversial for women's health. Testosterone is given in the form of shots, patches, creams, lozenges, pills, and even pellets injected under the skin. Intrinsa, a testosterone patch introduced by Proctor and Gamble to the FDA in 2004, promised hope for lackluster desire and falling testosterone levels in surgically postmenopausal women. The FDA blocked the progress of this treatment option, declaring insufficient long-term safety data to support approval even after more than three years of study. Many clinician and consumers view this as a male–female double standard in light of Viagra's approval for men in 1998. Viagra had only six months of clinical trials and possesses the potentially fatal risk for men who use Viagra with nitroglycerin medications. Research in women's sexual health is no doubt a decade behind research for men. My hope is that the bold lobby of baby-boomer women who are respected professionals and those passionate consumers will begin to right this wrong.

Let me share some of the other treatment choices to enhance sexual desire for women. Estratest, a combination of estrogen and testosterone first used for the treatment of hot flashes, has been recommended for some women to enhance desire. Although it is not FDA approved for low desire and thus remains off label, the ultimate decision remains between a woman and her provider. Beginning with low doses for a six-month period, monitoring potential adverse reactions and using the dose as prescribed may well provide women sexual zest. Adverse reactions to attend to are excess facial hair, oily skin, acne, and changes in voice quality. Another testosterone option is bioidentical testosterone compounded by a reliable pharmacy. The cream or gel can be applied to the inner thigh once a day. Some clinicians prescribe 2 percent testosterone gel, a thicker product, applied directly to the clitoris and surrounding areas about half an hour before bedtime each night. Again, if you do not respond within an 8- to 12-week period, recheck your free testosterone level and continue periodic testosterone levels to prevent a dangerous overabundance in the body.[24] Dr. William Regelson, author of *The Superhormone Promise,* argues that testosterone is the missing link in hormone therapy for women. He believes that adding testosterone to the hormonal "cocktail," even for a short period of time, helps women better tolerate estrogen and progesterone, restore sexual desire, improve energy, and promote a sense of well-being.[25]

Some members of the medical community remain suspect regarding androgen therapy for women and will not prescribe testosterone or other androgens. Some will not prescribe pills, which can increase the risk of liver toxicity or lower levels of high-density lipoprotein cholesterol (the good cholesterol) but will utilize the transdermal patch since this process bypasses the liver. Others having good success without marked negative side effects are prescribed but with protocols and ongoing testing. A reasonable approach to take until long-term studies are available is to obtain baseline testing, use lower doses, modulate the dose relative to results, educate consumers as to potential adverse effects, and perform ongoing testing to support continued dosing. A word of caution: testosterone therapy is not appropriate for childbearing-age women, as they produce sufficient androgens and an excess level can causes serious damage to a developing fetus. Finally, doses should be adjusted to an individual woman's needs, not a "one-size-fits-all" prescription. Talk to your health care provider if desire continues to plague your sense of sexual well-being and other conditions have been ruled out, as options to improve your sexual satisfaction are available.

DHEA therapy is new on the horizon for androgen treatment in women's health. It has been labeled in some articles as "the fountain of youth," news reports cite it as "the mother of all hormones," while others regard it as a fraud. My concern is that while the research does not yet provide long-term data, this potential supplement for women's health may get lost. DHEA is a precursor of testosterone. In other words, the body converts this steroid hormone into testosterone. It is secreted by the adrenal glands, two small glands that sit over the kidneys and that are responsible in part for production of at least 50 different hormones, including testosterone, estrogen, progesterone, cortisol, and epinephrine. A substantive level of DHEA helps the body recover from chronic stress and abuse of the adrenal glands that could lead to adrenal exhaustion or fatigue. Adrenal exhaustion is receiving more attention because women are continually attempting to cope with chronic stress. Adrenal glands cannot keep up with the emotional turmoil of life and attempts to juggle too many roles and responsibilities. Marcelle Pick, OB/GYN and nurse practitioner, acknowledges that some 99 percent of women in her practice have some indication of adrenal fatigue.[26]

The adrenals make very little DHEA in the first few years of life; by age six or seven, DHEA production begins. Then, by the mid-twenties, it is the most abundant hormone in circulation. A steady decline occurs in the mid-thirties so that by age 75, a woman may only have 20 percent of the DHEA that was in circulation at age 20. At all ages, men tend to have a higher DHEA level than women.

DHEA Can Help the Body Do the Following
- Neutralize cortisol (improving resistance to disease)
- Improve immune function
- Increase bone density
- Keep low-density lipoprotein cholesterol (the bad cholesterol) under control
- Maintain healthy sleep patterns
- Promote a sharp mind
- Assist in energy refueling
- Regulate lean muscle mass production
- Assist in "burning" fat
- Aid in memory and learning
- Assist in antiaging

DHEA is available in pill or cream form and can increase testosterone levels by one and a half to two times. Many clinicians prescribe as little as 5 mg two times a day to stabilize levels. Reasonable practice supports obtaining DHEA levels every three months while it is prescribed. It is little wonder that women enter their provider's office asking for a prescription after having seen a report, researched DHEA on the Internet, or talked to a friend using DHEA whose sexual interest has increased with an enhanced physical and mental satisfaction. Dr. Christiane Northrup recommends replenishing DHEA if both testosterone and DHEA are depleted. DHEA levels can be tested by blood or saliva; the most reliable results come from a daylong collection process to determine morning, midday, afternoon, and late night levels.[27]

Although DHEA can be obtained over the counter in most drugstores, I recommend working with a pharmaceutical-grade product to ensure the quality of the product for consumer use. When I prescribe DHEA cream, it is always with a compounding pharmacy that I have a relationship with and know their product grades. Before prescribing DHEA for an adrenally challenged woman, I encourage assessment of lifestyle, diet, and stress levels and instituting new interventions to maximize overall well-being.

Since the mind is the greatest stimulant for desire a romantic evening with your loved one, a diverse menu of sexual thoughts and foreplay to enrich the sexual connection would not hurt a thing. Sexual novels, sexual movies, sexual talk, sensual massage, and sexual fantasy can keep the spark ignited. Sexual desire is such an elusive component of sexuality that I have devoted an entire section of this chapter to help you unravel your own truth about desire and options to enhance it.

Sexual Arousal Disorders

Sexual arousal disorders occur when the mind and the genitals are out of sync. A woman may describe an absence of or markedly diminished feelings of sexual arousal and pleasure from any type of sexual stimulation. This category of sexual disorder is a subjective component since a woman can be aroused by sexual stimulation yet have a marked loss in the intensity of genital response, even orgasm. Planning that sexual adventure, watching a sexy movie, or reading an erotic novel, can stimulate excitement and bring the "wanting" to the surface. Your heart rate increases, breath quickens, breasts begin to swell, nipples become erect, muscles in the body tense, and then the genitals respond. Blood flows to the pelvic region, the clitoris swells and becomes more sensitive, vaginal lubrication increases, and the body is in a state of readiness. But what if you "want" to engage your arousal network— the mind is willing but the body is weak? When pleasurable sensations are blocked, it is important to rule out interference from medications such as beta blockers for high blood pressure or drugs to decrease anxiety, such as selective serotonin reuptake inhibitors (SSRIs), which diminish the sexual tension needed to complete the arousal circuit. Zestra, a botanical topical formula, can be used to increase vaginal sensitivity.[28] ArginMax, another topical, contains the amino acid L-arginine, which stimulates blood flow to the vulva and clitoris, thus activating the arousal mechanism. Some of my patients state that even if they are not as aroused, applying Zestra helps the body and mind become more responsive.

Dr. Robert Greene, a renowned hormone specialist, recommends bioidentical estrogen therapy for arousal disorders. These products dilate the blood vessels in the vulva much like Viagra for male erectile disorder dilates vessels in the penis. Estring a vaginal ring is a safe low-dose bioidentical estrogen that is inserted and left in place for three months at a time. For a higher dose of bioidentical estrogen with a vaginal delivery, Femring is another option and, like Estring, can be inserted, left in for three month, and changed after that time frame. Vagifem, another bioidentical estrogen product in tablet form, is inserted into the vagina by an applicator every other day.[29] Another option to heighten arousal is the Eros Clitoral Therapy Device. The handheld suction device placed on the genital area increases engorgement in the clitoris without side effects. It is recommended for use three to five times a week as part of a couple's foreplay activity. Eros is by prescription only and is cited to improve genital sensations, clitoral sensations, lubrication, and orgasm and is FDA approved for arousal disorders.[30]

"About 20 percent of women between the ages of eighteen and fifty-nine experience problems with sexual arousal. The number jumps to 40 percent for women going through their menopausal transition without hormone therapy," notes Dr. Greene.[31] Women frustrated by decrease of their arousal need not suffer the loss of pleasure. Talk to your health care provider, share your concerns, and ask about the options available to you. Often referral to a certified sex therapist can identify the inhibitors affecting arousal and other forms of sexual dysfunction. The American Association of Sexuality Educators, Counselors and Therapists provides a listing of certified therapists in your area (see http://www.aasect.org).

Orgasmic Disorders

Orgasmic disorders are often not a new complaint for women. Far too many young women, childbearing women, and seniors struggle with the inability to experience orgasm. And every year, probably 80 percent of my client cases enter treatment for sexual desire disorders (which I refer to as "discrepancy of desire"), 10 percent complain of orgasmic disorders, and 10 percent sexual pain disorders. Women's orgasmic disorder has recently been redefined by the International Consensus Study as follows: "Despite the self-report of high sexual arousal/excitement, there is either lack of orgasm, markedly diminished intensity of orgasmic sensations or marked delay of orgasm from any kind of stimulation."[32] In fact, the majority of women do not experience orgasm from intercourse alone; they require extended clitoral or vaginal stimulation to intensify arousal and move to orgasm.

Anorgasmia is the inability to achieve orgasm/climax during intercourse. It affects approximately 24 to 37 percent of women, reports R. Rosen.[33] Primary orgasmic disorder refers to a woman who has never experienced orgasm through any means of stimulation, including self-stimulation. Secondary orgasmic disorder is diagnosed when the woman has attained orgasm in the past but is currently nonorgasmic. Orgasm is a brief event on the average 25 seconds for men and 17 seconds for women.[34] The menopausal woman's time frame is even less.

Anorgasmia May Result from the Following Multiple Factors

- Fatigue
- Depression
- Worry
- Anxiety
- Stress
- Guilt
- Fear of painful intercourse
- Fear of pregnancy
- Prescription drugs
- Medical conditions that affect nerves in the pelvis
- Chronic illness
- Hormone disorders
- Use of alcohol
- Conflict with a partner
- An unpleasant setting

The hormone–brain connection has more responsibility for orgasm than the sexual attraction or technique of a couple. Low estrogen and testosterone levels can hinder an orgasm, thus leaving a menopausal woman at risk for fewer orgasms or orgasms with less intensity than she previously experienced. Other hormones involved in the orgasmic process are oxytocin, prolactin, phenylethylamine (PEA), and the stress hormones cortisol, epinephrine, and norephinephrine. Women in a tense state at the onset of sex challenge the orgasmic process since the tension necessary to trigger an orgasm may already be at maximum threshold. One technique to offset this problem is to learn and apply relaxation techniques and a peaceful state of mind as you enter sexual play. PEA hormones produce a chemical feeling of euphoria at orgasm. That "runner's high" you feel during 20 minutes of vigorous exercise is very much like the response your body feels from the release of PEA.

With orgasm, some hormones that have peaked during arousal return to baseline, while other hormones rise and produce the feeling of warmth and connection after orgasm. Testosterone and the stress hormones that propelled you to orgasm now slow. Oxytocin is the hormone responsible for uterine contractions during orgasm and a sense of connection between lovers. Oxytocin rises after orgasm and remains elevated for several hours. Couples often comment after having sex, "That was so good. Why don't we do this more often?" I now have more appreciation for oxytocin and its hormonal function. Prolactin consistently rises during orgasm and remains elevated for some time after orgasm. It may just be the hormone responsible for ending the sexual cascade of pleasure. And for some with an elevated prolactin level, it can result in a reduction of sexual drive or libido.

I have described the hormonal interactions responsible for orgasm. But without a doubt, the major trigger for orgasms in women remains stimulation of the clitoris. Until 30 years ago Dr. Freud's proposal that vaginal orgasms were the only true orgasm prevailed. Today, clinicians describe three types of orgasm: vaginal, clitoral, and combination. Clitoral orgasms are the norm, and some women can provoke orgasm without clitoris stimulation or even without touch. These responses are less common but worth mentioning. I had a client years ago with persistent genital arousal—a throbbing, pulsation in her genitals without sexual interest or stimulation. Orgasm did not relieve the sensations of arousal; in fact, hours after orgasm, she described a fullness in her genitals and ongoing vasocongestion. Clinically, we now know that this is not as rare a condition as once believed, and treatment can be quite a challenge.

How many women have made the proclamation, "Honey, I do not have to have an orgasm each and every time we are sexual to enjoy the pleasure and connection we share."? Indeed, for many women, the closeness, emotional connection, and sexual excitement may be as far as they can travel on that particular sexual journey. A woman's orgasm can be stalled when she is not in a positive mind-set or when she is fatigued, angry, anxious, or hurt. When a woman is satisfied overall with her sexual relationship but periodically does not reach orgasm, I would not describe her as having orgasmic disorder. I caution couples not to let infrequent orgasms become a stumbling block in their relationship if the overall satisfaction is present.

Beverly Whipple, sexual researcher, nurse, and colleague in AASECT, has long been a champion for women's sexual health. Her book *The Science of Orgasm* explores the complex biological process leading to orgasm. For those women or couples wanting to explore the G-spot, her book *The G Spot and Other Discoveries about Human Sexuality* is a must read.[35] The G-spot is discussed later in this chapter.

In my private practice, a few significant causes create an orgasmic disconnect. Negative attitudes about sex or one's partner are the most pronounced. Often the lack of information or negative messages in childhood create the sexual block; educating a woman about her body, working through the negative messages, and creating a new mind-set for sexual well-being provides a new foundation for sexuality. Sexual abuse or rape incidents from the past are another significant barrier. When a woman comes for sex therapy with the complaint of never having an orgasm, often it may be the first time she has shared her hurt and her story of abuse. Lack of emotional closeness with a partner or significant relationship barriers can also build the orgasmic disconnect. The boredom in the bedroom that prevents her from reaching those higher levels of arousal or her man's absence of attention to her needs for stimulation or variety are other complaints I hear all too often. Thirty-five to 50 percent of women report in surveys that they experience orgasms infrequently or are dissatisfied with how often they reach orgasm. And statistics now indicate that from 50 to 70 percent of women do not have vaginal orgasms from penetration alone.

Treatment options for orgasmic disorders begin with a physical assessment, and medications commonly given for depression and anxiety—the SSRIs, such as Prozac, Zoloft, and Paxil—can inhibit orgasm. If you need to be on these medications, one option is to talk with your provider about adding Wellbutrin. This addition increases the dopamine action in the brain, thus enhancing libido. Chocolate with high cocoa content can boost the euphoria-inducing chemical PEA. It is always fun to prescribe dark chocolate as part of foreplay for my clients. I am, however, a bit more cautious in promoting a glass or two of wine to boost testosterone and decrease inhibitions. Kegel exercises have long been part of the treatment plan to improve the frequency and intensity if orgasms.

Hormonal treatment to balance estrogen and testosterone and thus enhance orgasmic flow should also be considered. Bioidentical estrogen in the form of a patch, gel, or vaginal ring will also positively impact orgasm and support testosterone levels. Bioidentical testosterone applied to the skin via patch at 300 mcg/day minimizes risk factors and promotes the frequency and intensity of orgasm. Testosterone gel is another option for orgasmic health. The plan details a slow process of testosterone gel 2 mg/day applied to the inner thighs and gradually increased by 1 mg every 10 to 12 weeks to a maximum of 5 mg based on the woman's orgasmic response. Unfortunately, testosterone therapy for orgasmic disorder remains off label.[36] It is important to remember there are so many variables related to orgasm and the menopausal woman that testosterone is not the only or even the best choice for the majority of women. The good news is that options await you; do not stop if one provider is unresponsive to your questions. Talk to your primary care provider and friends about approachable clinicians or contact professional organizations for potential referrals, such as AASECT.

Sexual Pain Disorders

Sexual pain disorders are unfortunately very common and not well understood. Dyspareunia, vaginismus, atropic vaginitis, vulvar vestibultis, and vulvodynia are the most common. "Persistent or recurrent pain with attempted or complete vaginal entry and/or penile vaginal intercourse" is the most current definition of dypareunia by the International Consultation Panel.[37] Structural or other physical conditions should be ruled out before the diagnosis is given.

A woman often describes anticipation or fear of pain and avoidance of sexual contact. When pain begins on entry of the penis, it is often caused by inadequate lubrication, requiring more sexual stimulation and time for arousal. *Dyspareunia* is estimated to affect 14.4 percent of women annually, according to the National Health and Social Life Survey, while vaginismus affects 15 to 17 percent of women entering sex therapy clinics.[38] *Vaginismus* is defined as "persistent difficulties to allow vaginal entry of a penis, a finger, and/or any object, despite the woman's expressed wish to do so. There is often (phobic) avoidance, involuntary pelvic muscle contraction and anticipation/fear of the experience of pain. Structural or other physical abnormalities must be ruled out or addressed."[39]

Other pain-related sexual disorders can be due to structural conditions, hormonal imbalance, an impatient partner, premature lovemaking following surgery, inflammation, infections, genital mutilation, trauma, vestibulitis, surgery for prolapse or incontinence, and endometriosis. "Vulvodynia is vulva discomfort in the absence of gross anatomical or neurological findings," as defined by the International Society for the Study of Vulvar Disease. Women complain of burning, stinging, irritation, and rawness. In 1987, E. G. Friedrich published the criteria for vulvadynia. What was once thought to be a rare disease now affects 16 percent of the population when compared with other chronic diseases, such as low back pain (52%), fibromyalgia (2%), and diabetes (7%). The highest incidence is with women younger than age 25. In the past year in my practice alone, the number of women referred to me for sex therapy with vulvadynia has tripled.[40]

The most common disorder for menopausal women is atrophic vaginitis (vaginal atrophy), or thinning of the vaginal tissue and inflammation. It can take one to three years of estrogen loss for atrophy to be pronounced, even though early signs of wasting can begin in perimenopause. The chronic burning described by some women may be initiated by herpes simplex virus, yeast infections, an imbalance of the normal vaginal bacteria, or bacterial vaginosis. Cultures can rule out the variables and establish the appropriate treatment. When sexual pain continues without therapeutic interventions, a couple risks serious dissatisfaction in the intimate relationship, including unconsummated marriages, resentment, and even male erectile dysfunction after repeated rejection or unsuccessful attempts at partnering.

Treatment begins with medical assessment for physical concerns and infection and evaluation of the pelvic floor. Encouragement of adequate foreplay and stimulation can enhance lubrication. The use of water-soluble lubricant like K-Y jelly, Astroglide, and silicone products may be helpful. Vaseline should not be used as a sexual lubricant, as it can increase vaginal infections. Vaginal or oral estrogen in various forms—pills, creams, rings (Estring), vaginal moisturizers, and lubricants—can be prescribed to assist the woman with vaginal atrophy. Women using estrogen or testosterone topical creams are encouraged to protect others from accidental exposure by applying creams to body parts that are not exposed to touch. Apply creams to the inner thighs after sexual activity or bathing to prevent low-dose exposure to others. Assessment and intervention with physical therapy for increasing blood flow to the vagina and healing the effective area with pelvic floor exercises and biofeedback, which is a computer-assisted device that measures muscle activity and teaches women how to contract and properly relax the muscles, has been invaluable for my clients. Use of vaginal dilators to desensitize the woman for penetration and promote comfort is also beneficial for vaginismus. Therapy combining sex education, working through fears and avoidance issues, resolving relationship resentments, and including the partner in treatment is very successful when treated by a specialist in sex therapy.

I am often asked by women without partners what to do for their genital and sexual health. The old adage "if you don't use it, you will lose it" is very true regarding women's sexual health. The vagina needs regular blood flow to maintain the integrity of the tissues, and the clitoris can become less responsive to touch if it is ignored for periods of time. I encourage women without partners or with partners who are not engaged in regular sexual activity to regularly stimulate the vagina and genitals by self-pleasuring (masturbation) either manually or with a vibrator. Kegel exercises are very helpful to maintain vaginal health. Vaginal exercises with vaginal barbells, dilators, weights, and cones keep the vagina stretched and help prevent atrophy. These can be purchased through some of the popular Web sites cited in Appendix D. Lubricate the barbell or dilator, insert it half way into the vagina, and then squeeze the vaginal muscles around the bar for 5 to 10 minutes at a time. This exercise practiced two or three times a week is very beneficial for vaginal health. If you have trouble with the Kegel exercises or other vaginal workouts, see a physical therapist trained in women's health with a specialty in pelvic floor training. Your gynecologist or other provider can easily make the referral.

STRATEGIES FOR TREATMENT OF SEXUAL DYSFUNCTIONS

Interventions without Medications

- Communicate about sexual needs and partner concerns
- Increase the time for stimulation
- Experiment with erotic toys, lotions, sexual fantasies, and vibrators
- Explore sensual massage
- Use water-based lubricants and moisturizers

- Focus on sexual activity other than intercourse, such as oral sex, mutual masturbation, sensual massage, and self-pleasuring
- Increase the variety of sexual play moving beyond the normal routine
- Seek counseling or sex therapy

Interventions with Medication
- Androgen therapy: testosterone and DHEA
- Topical or oral estrogen and progesterone therapy
- Modify doses and types of medications that can affect sexual function (with physician input): antidepressants

SEX AFTER HYSTERECTOMY, CHEMOTHERAPY, AND RADIATION

Induced menopause through surgery, chemotherapy, or radiation can affect not only the emotional and physical state of women but also their concerns and fears regarding their sexual health and abilities. Emotional concerns include loss of fertility, mortality, side effects from the procedure, recurrence of disease, and loss of sexual function. Women are encouraged to examine their own fears, talk to their partner, and relate these concerns to their health care provider. However, recent studies show that mental health and overall quality of life improve for most women after hysterectomy. They no longer are bothered by ongoing pain or excessive bleeding and can reclaim their spontaneity and sexual pleasure. The Maine Women's Study of women undergoing hysterectomy for benign disease and dyspareunia showed improvement of interest in and enjoyment of sexual activity one year after surgery.[41]

Other studies suggest an adverse effect with the removal of both ovaries on libido and orgasmic response. This may be due to a decline in androgens (testosterone) postsurgery. If there is an option of retaining the ovaries for women undergoing hysterectomy, the majority of physicians support leaving them to continue the production of androgens and circulating estrogen unless there is an estrogen-sensitive form of breast, ovarian, or uterine cancer.

Cancer therapies with chemotherapy or radiation produce a physical and emotional risk for a woman's well-being. The pain and discomfort, change in body image, fear of death, apprehension over sexual function, and impact on the family are but a few of the struggles after diagnosis. Women need not only an approachable clinician for questions but also an empathetic educator for the process. Many times the fatigue, nausea, hair loss, and alteration in body image when addressed early in the process can short-circuit mood disorders. Therapy for a woman and her family can often be of help when emotional or physical issues overwhelm them. Agents may irritate the vagina and the uterus lining, leaving it dry and easily inflamed by sexual friction. Some women experience no change in their ovary function after chemotherapy. For others, the ovaries shut down, and desire is dampened because of a drop in estrogen and testosterone. Whether ovarian dysfunction is a permanent problem or a temporary change in desire only time will tell.

Pelvic radiation may cause itching, burning, dryness, and tenderness during treatment and persist for weeks afterward. The walls of the vagina can be tender to the touch and fibrous, lose elasticity, and become thin, fragile, and more prone to sores and ulcers. Radiation can even shorten the vagina, making intercourse painful or impossible. Most women can resume intercourse within a few weeks after treatment. Some women benefit greatly by hormone therapy, which can restore the healthy lining of the vagina, as well as sexual desire, with circulating hormones. Risks and benefits must always be discussed between a woman and her health care provider. Hormone therapy is usually not recommended for those with an estrogen-sensitive form of breast, ovarian, or uterine cancer. Zestra, a biotanical vaginal stimulant, contains no estrogen products and has been very effective for women wanting to boost the sexual sensations in their genitals and awaken desire. Determining what types of stimulation and sexual play a couple want to explore often can reconnect sexual lives after surgery or chemotherapy.

UNCOVERING STALL-OUTS IN SEXUAL DEVELOPMENT

Let's revisit Lexie, the woman from the beginning of the chapter complaining of a lukewarm sexual connection with her husband and unsatisfying orgasms. After several couples' sessions to assess their relationship factors and several more to work on the old resentments and redefine a new sexual pathway, Lexie and I began individual therapy sessions. Lexie's sexual development had stalled out during preadolescence, leaving her with many misconceptions about sex and a silent sexual voice.

June, age 53, entered therapy when her daughter turned 12. June waited to have children until age 34. She chose to spend her early adulthood developing her law practice, but when the biological clock clamored in her head at age 31, she began her quest for motherhood. Unfortunately, her body was not in agreement with her timetable; conception took longer than she had planned. As her daughter approached adolescence, she became aware of her uneasiness regarding sex not only in her relationship with Jim, her husband, but also in her attempts to talk with Ann Marie, her daughter. "I do not want to repeat the sexual legacy with Ann Marie. My parents were not affectionate. They were civil with one another, but very little warmth seemed to exist between them. They gave me negative messages about sex. 'Good girls don't date at 14. You will get pregnant if a boy even touches you. And sex is all they want so do not trust them,'" she remarked tearfully one session. These two stories are not unusual for women entering sex therapy. June's anxiety over trying to talk with her daughter about sex thrust her into treatment. She was determined not to let her daughter negotiate the turbulent waters of sexual development with negative messages. "Where do I begin?" was her cry.

Lately, a new group of women in their fifties and sixties have made their way into sex therapy—postmenopausal women feeling better with the absence of hot flashes, finally sleeping, and feeling a little spunky in the evening as they nestle in for the night with their partner. Many were also uneducated for the role of a fully developed sexual woman who knows what she likes, can ask that her needs be met, and is comfortable trying new erotic play. This later group wants to be self-reflective; they have the time and energy to explore sexuality, fewer demands are placed on them by family, and generally their professional world is stable. "Why can't these be my best years? After all, I can live another 30 to 40 years and not have to worry about periods or pregnancy. And I like who I am, for the most part, and I know sex can be better. I just need some help to figure it out." How I enjoy these women and the self-discovery.

Sexual development can be stalled out by numerous factors: messages from parents, peer group pressure, sexual play that is shamed, sexual abuse, trauma during a first experience with sex, and dissatisfaction with body image. When is the first time you can remember receiving the message that your sexual thoughts, sexual feelings, and sexual behaviors were not okay? Do those messages continue to rule your sex life today? Women can begin the uncovering process and create positive messages about sex when they review early messages from parents, religious beliefs, and influences from peer groups. Lexie was told that being sexual would make her a "bad girl," and since her older sister had disappointed her parents with her sexual free spirit, Lexie chose to be the "good girl." Some women are blocked sexually if they were discovered masturbating and shamed terribly. I have worked with a number of midlife women sharing for the first time a sexual trauma or sexual abuse that held them hostage from sexual freedom. Gently uncovering traumas and changing negative self-talk, ranging from "I do not deserve to feel sexual pleasure" to the antidote "I am a sexual woman free from the past and choosing to experience pleasure," engages a woman in a present-day belief system. If the pain remains potent today, making it difficult to engage a new sexual spirit, one that fits the woman you have become, I hope you will consider working with a therapist to unlock the issues and heal.

Factors Influencing Sexual Development

- Messages from parents
- Religious beliefs
- Peer group influences
- Media

- Sexual play and curiosity
- Abuse experiences
- Traumas in sexual relationships

Basic principles are addressed with these courageous women early in treatment. First, we discuss a physical exam to rule out any physiological problems. Second, we focus on her current sexual messages and attitudes and then education to reframe messages and establish a new foundation for sexuality. Third, and probably the most novel for the majority of women, is the message that she is responsible for her own pleasure and sexuality. A woman who shows up for sex out of "duty" and without her own needs, even if her needs have less intensity than a partner's, is doing herself and the relationship a disservice by having sex. Promoting the mind-set that this is your body, your sensual and sexual self, and it is your opportunity to "own your sexuality" for yourself first and then choose when and how you want to "share" your pleasure with your partner is a critical step in recovering from sexual stall-outs. Fourth, a woman needs to be educated about sexual stimulation and response. If you have never explored your own body and its erogenous zones, how can you direct the stimulation you need from your partner? Self-pleasuring for many women seems wrong or dirty. Moving beyond that block can take the therapy process into a new land of sensual discovery. A "treasure hunt" takes on new meaning for this voyager. Later in this chapter, I provide the Treasure Hunt Exercise. Sexual stimulation is only part of the equation for successful pleasuring. What if the response to sexual stimuli is blocked, cut off, or purposefully denied? In my experience, the sexual process and any potential for satisfying lovemaking will end if a woman "chooses not to respond." Many homework sessions are spent on this fourth principle. Finally, it is critical for couples to realize that they must verbally and nonverbally guide their partner in providing them with the stimulation that provokes those higher levels of arousal. Guiding a hand, moaning with pleasure, sharing your fantasy for the evening, and verbalizing the type of touch, the firmness, and the location are all certain to provide the excitement you need and will enrich the experience for both of you.

Treatment Principles for Sexual Stall-Outs
- Have a physical exam to rule out physical problems
- Uncover sexual messages, attitudes and reeducate
- Accept responsibility for pleasure and sexuality
- Learn pathways to sexual stimulation and response
- Verbally and nonverbally guide the partner

The second component that can inhibit the sexual person a woman wants to be is satisfaction with *body image.* Eighty percent of women are dissatisfied with their appearance, and more than 45 percent of women are on a diet at any given time. Why are so many dissatisfied with their bodies? It isn't just the "body beautiful" world we live in that extols women who are thin, busty, and long legged and who glide as they walk. In order for these images to have meaning to you, you have to make comparisons of yourself with others and value those comparisons. At this age, how nice not to expect a flat stomach, pert breasts, and slender hips. In fact, the average American woman is five feet four inches tall, weighs 145 pounds, and wears a size 12.[42] Women can be more comfortable with their bodies as they celebrate the accomplishments of years past, the paths they have taken, the children they carried into the world, and the fact that their identity is not based on one distinct factor. Learning to appreciate your body as it is and valuing body parts is a lifelong process for the seasoned siren within.

Body image is an ever-changing picture. Remember how you looked as a young girl? Adolescence is a tricky junction in life and carries many changes: hormones, breast development, genital awakening, acne, and the onset of intense sexual feelings. What was your comfort in adolescence with your body? Young adulthood becomes an opportunity to merge the adolescent image with the preferred adult image. Did you negotiate the merger with ease or with conflict? Womanhood and motherhood can be a new time for discovery. For some, motherhood creeps in before the woman has an opportunity to be fully formed.

The mature woman enters the transition into menopause gifted with her past body image and the ever-evolving new body image. My work with women and body image has grown over the years into a more comprehensive model. Body image is more than the physical mass. It includes the way you dress or your personal style, hairstyle, and the voice quality you project. You may want to take a few minutes to explore the first part of body image with the Body Image Exercise in the "Strategies" section later in this chapter. This exercise gives you an opportunity to instill more confidence in the image you possess.

A second level of body image investigation involves appreciation of your body parts. When was the last time you really looked at your body—not the "clothes on" investigation but exploring the shape, size, and symmetry of all your body parts? Take the time and turn to the Body Appreciation Exercise in the "Strategies" section later in this chapter. It will only take 20 minutes of your time, but the payoff will be an enhancement of the image you hold of "the mature woman" of today and will prepare you for the next level: your sexual investigation.

Women who have explored their genitals and felt comfortable with them and comfortable with genital odor are often the woman with a positive body image who is able to experience heightened levels of arousal, move to orgasm, and have an enjoyable sexual relationship with themselves and a partner. This observation was validated by the work of Dr. Laura Berman at the Berman

Center, which conducted a nationwide study of more than 2,500 women ages 18 and over to determine the impact of genital self-image on their sexual response and satisfaction. A second finding of the study related to how body image and genital odor impact a woman's genital self-image. Women were asked if they felt comfortable or ashamed with their genitals. Berman's results showed that "women with more positive genital self-images were found to have more sexual desire and better sexual response."[43]

Berman has been generous in giving permission for me to share her *Genital Image Scale* in the "Strategies" section later this chapter.[44] Her book *The Passion Prescription: Ten Weeks to Your Best Sex-Ever* is a frequent homework assignment for my clients. The concise information, interesting exercises, and the "Guy's Guide" at the end of each chapter are very helpful in recharging a couple's sex life.

What is your comfort with your genitals? Have you taken a mirror to examine "down there"? Being familiar with your sexual anatomy is a woman's responsibility in maintaining sexual health. You wouldn't own and drive a car for a decade or more and not know where to pour oil or how to inflate a low tire. We often begin the self-discovery by dispelling language myths. The *vagina* is not the correct name for all the genital structures. *Vulva* describes the external anatomy consisting of the labia (lips), clitoris, and other structures, including the vagina. Some compare the shape of the vagina to a banana that curves upward toward the back. It can measure from five to seven inches long and expands during arousal and childbirth. The first third of the vaginal opening possesses many nerve endings; it is pleasurable when massaged and leads to the *G-spot* (see Figure 8.1).

The existence of the G-spot and its exploration have long been debated. First, it does exist. Second, if you have not explored this tiny spot with its rich sensations, make a date to explore it soon. The drawing provided helps with its general location. Now, lay on your back and insert a finger into your vagina on the anterior wall about the 12:00 position. The spongy bump, about the texture of the tip of your nose and about the size of a pea, is the G-spot. Rub gently at first until the pea changes into the size of a quarter. The sensations can continue to rise and create a very pleasant feeling and, for some, an intense orgasm (see Figure 8.2).

Educating women and their partner about the pleasure zone known as the *clitoris* and its similarity to the penis can be eye opening. Did you know that the clitoris, with all its structures, can measure up to four inches long? The structure of the clitoris is not simply the soft fold of skin (the clitoral hood) and fleshy knob covered by the hood that when massaged can produce sensual feelings and orgasm. It extends internally into the pelvic region another two to three inches and is made up of the same erectile tissue as the penis. And

Figure 8.1
Female Sexual Anatomy

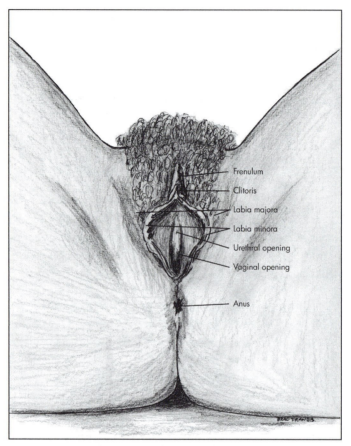

Frenulum
Clitoris
Labia majora
Labia minora
Urethral opening
Vaginal opening
Anus

Artist: George Brad Francis.

like the penis, the clitoris, all four inches of it, when stimulated, fills with blood and increases in size, creating intense feelings of arousal. Even though the intensity of clitoral stimulation can change (and for some menopausal women that can be a decrease of sensation), the clitoris remains the primary trigger for female orgasm. Tune in to the pleasing sensations when your clitoris is stimulated either manually or orally and share whether direct or indirect contact feels the best. If the clitoris becomes overstimulated, speak up, as a partner cannot read your mind. Remember that every sexual encounter is different—sensations are different, and the orgasm is different—and that you are the transmitter of clitoral pleasure by your moans or your words or moving your partner's hand to a more pleasurable location.

Figure 8.2
Female Anatomy with G-Spot

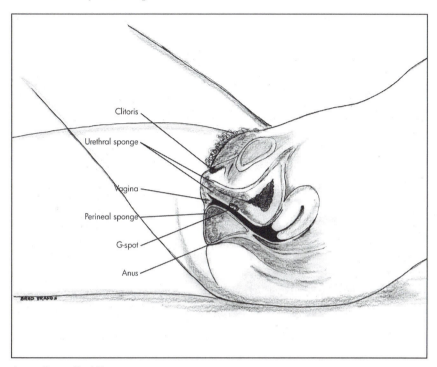

Artist: George Brad Francis.

Sensual touch of your entire body is an important exercise to uncover the range and intensity of arousal you are able to experience. The Touch Yourself Sensate Focus Touch Exercise can be found in the "Strategies" section later in this chapter. This exercise comes from the work of Barbara Keesling, Ph.D., author and sex therapist.[45] Women like Lexie who are unfamiliar with the arousal process have benefited from this exercise. It is important for women to understand that the arousal process takes about 8 to 10 minutes for moderate levels of arousal to build and for some women more like 30 minutes to achieve intensity for orgasm to become triggered. Lexie learned from this full body touch exercise that her standard arousal level with Ben was low or level 1. She discovered that when her face, breasts, and inner thighs were gently stroked by Ben, before heading to the genitals she could relax and experience intense arousal (level 3). They developed a richer land of erotic touch only after Lexie experimented with this exercise over a two-week period. Do not miss the opportunity to savor the pleasure and learn your levels of arousal.

FACTORS OF SEXUAL SATISFACTION

To determine a woman's level of sexual satisfaction and any inhibiting factors, therapists generally evaluate at least five other features, assessing her satisfaction with the relationship outside the bedroom, the elements of attraction to her partner, arousal components, the orgasmic process, and satisfaction, or "afterglow." My assessment tool is composed of a list of questions for women. I begin with the early influences, such as messages from a parent, and then incorporate present-day circumstances:

- Are you satisfied with your relationship outside the bedroom?
- How attracted are you to your partner?
- What inhibiting feelings or thoughts interfere with your level of desire?
- Do you have sex in places other than the bedroom?
- Are you turned on by movies or books?
- How satisfied are you with foreplay?
- Are there any barriers to sexual satisfaction?

Arousal (Heightened Levels of Sexual Excitement)

- Do you have a change in arousal?
- Do you know what is responsible for the change in arousal?
- Do you feel aroused when your partner touches your body?
- Do sensations build? What feels the best?
- Do distracting feelings or thoughts stop sensations?
- Have you tried vibrators, toys, or lotions to increase the pleasure?
- Do you feel comfortable talking to your partner about the kinds of stimulation you like?
- Does your vagina become dry with arousal? What do you do?

Orgasm (Intense Physical Pleasure Accompanied by Quick Muscle Contractions in the Pelvis and a General Euphoric State)

- Have you had an orgasm?
- What do you do to reach high levels of arousal for orgasm?
- Do thoughts or feelings inhibit orgasm?
- Do you expect to have an orgasm each time?
- Are you satisfied with orgasm?

Afterglow (The Sense of Satisfaction and Closeness after Orgasmic Release)

- What do you like to do after sex?
- Do you spend adequate time with afterglow to enjoy it fully?

Lexie took advantage of Ben's support and delight in her sexual growth to venture into the land of pleasure. She explored old corroded sexual messages, her body, and her style of dress and took a huge leap (risk) to refashion a new identity and playful spirit for their relationship. The sexual assessment questions and body awareness exercises allowed her to move at her own pace into the land of pleasure. My role became more permission giving, role modeling, and encouraging her discovery. As a couple, they are playfully engaging each other, safely investigating toys, and making sex a comfortable priority in their lives.

RELATIONSHIP REALIGNMENT

Marriage is not immune to the changes that menopause creates for a woman and those she loves. Even solid relationships that have weathered the early years, established a career, and nurtured the connection between partners can find this stage of life extremely challenging. People in general are not that fond of change. If you have embraced "change" over the years and made change a traveling companion, you have an advantage. Just consider the emotional and physical changes of menopause: body image adjustments, a cascade of hormonal upheaval, launching children, partnership needs, and retirement.

Christiane Northrup, M.D., suggests that divorce or a heart attack are not the only options at this junction of life. "Rather, in order to bring your relationship into alignment with your rewired brain, you and your significant other must be willing to take the time, and spend the energy, to resolve old issues and set new ground rules for the years that lie ahead."[46] The rewired brain will not let you forget that time is at the heart of your change process. Each of the symptoms of menopause that challenges you has its own cycle of time. The good news is that you do not have to endure it forever. If hot flashes, night sweats, and nights of two-hour awakenings disrupt your well-being and sanity, contact an approachable clinician for help.

I met Sarah in my office early one morning. She sat on the sofa fanning her face, neck, and chest. Her cheeks were flushed, and perspiration beaded on her hairline. "I have been trying to deal with these flushes since my hysterectomy in 2004; it is now 2008, and if I do not do something soon, my patient husband will leave, and the tender thread that holds my sanity in place will snap." Sarah has shared her concerns with her family practice physician without relief of her symptoms. They tried one hormone cocktail over a year ago without success. But the reality is that a vast number of physicians are not specialists in the world of hormone replacement. We collected saliva samples two weeks previously; her results were in and reflected the need for progesterone and help for her adrenal fatigue. No wonder she slept only two hours at a time. Her midnight cortisol level was markedly elevated and progesterone below low normal.

Sarah and her husband just returned from celebrating their twenty-fifth wedding anniversary in Key West. How sad that their romantic rendezvous bumped up against low desire, fatigue from little sleep, and frequent flashing. Hopefully, next year's anniversary will surpass this year's by miles.

What about couples with unresolved relationship problems—problems that include past hurts, resentments, an imbalance of power, and sacrifices made that now are no longer tolerable? Each of these problems can send a couple into a downward spiral at any junction in the life of a relationship; menopause can hasten the deliberation as a woman's voice may be stronger now. Issues that went underground to protect a relationship are now fair game for resolution. Some of my favorite client work—and sometimes the most difficult—is approached from this arena in therapy.

A woman who overfunctions for decades to preserve a family system and protect an emotionally absent husband is at risk of losing that role during midlife. She is little prepared when the man she cared for in spite of his emotional neglect for her and the children wanders into a midlife crisis and announces his intent to leave. These stories often involve another woman whose arms are waiting. How does the overfunctioning wife who cared for the children, tended the social calendar, and preserved the family integrity manage the loss? Rivers of tears are shed, weight is lost, and people at work rise to her aid—factors of coping with the deep loss. The fortunate few enter therapy—they think to resolve the loss—and they "find themselves" in the process. Bold women uncover the overfunctioning and pledge not to follow that path again in any relationship. Finding themselves, meaningful relationships, and sometimes a new love are benefits of the uncovering process.

Couples determined to resolve past hurts and journey into their golden years together have taught me much about loyalty to vows taken and the integrity of the soul. These indeed are soulful people. One couple comes to mind, a couple having spent more than 40 years together growing and living a full life in the majority of areas. Helen grew up with a critical mother whose sense of caution created intense anxiety in Helen. Her sexuality became dormant because of the fear-filled messages she carried in her head. David, a loving, understanding man who adored Helen, tried his best to love and live without a sexual connection. His artistic nature became his sexual outlet until in his sixties it no longer dampened the desire for Helen. A very cautious couple entered my office that winter day, a couple who eventually taught me as much about love, tenacity, growth, and understanding as I taught them about sexuality. Helen ventured into the world of sexuality, a world whose door had been sealed more than 30 years ago. She bravely challenged the old sexual messages and even told and showed him how she wanted to be pleasured. Then the challenge fell to David: after decades of suppressed desire, he had to learn how to transform the artistic desire into intimacy with Helen. At the heart of intimacy are vulnerability and the desire to self-disclose—not an easy transition when you have shut down the vulnerability to need and want to be sexual. David's sensitive spirit and moments of insight helped him with the transition. Then sexual performance caught him by surprise. A 68-year-old man's health status and medications can greatly impact his erectile performance in spite of a resurgence of desire. Testosterone therapy was an option after a weak response to Viagra. Thirty years of absent sexual contact does not doom a couple for a lifetime. Couples willing to identify barriers, own their part in the disconnect, and patiently work through the resentments can obtain a new intimate connection.

Relationship realignment opens the opportunities to examine previous needs for one another, both personal and professional needs, and to structure an inviting future. Balancing your personal and professional lives—the need for "alone" time and for exploring a new passion and deciding if the career path you have taken is where you choose to remain, perhaps moving from fast-tracker to mentor. I see this as a private investigation, sometimes pursued alone and sometimes with professional help. But what if one member of the couple is contemplating these factors and the other is content with the status quo? Bitterness, anger, and distancing may result for the unfortunate couple unable to share their awareness and gain understanding, if not acceptance. Silence is the deal breaker. Even a good fight is better than silence and disregard for one's new insight.

ROMANCING THE MIDLIFE RELATIONSHIP

In today's marriages, in which people work long hours, travel extensively, and juggle career needs with family needs, couples find more forces tugging at the relationship than ever before. Modern marriages are battered by the demands of the workplace and family, changing community values, self-care struggles, retirement plans, and a host of other issues.

The ease of divorce and changing attitudes about the permanence of marriage have themselves become centrifugal forces. Understanding the power that each member of a couple possesses and learning how to balance the power and not abuse it has helped countless couples step away from the cliff of divorce and recommit with passion and romance. Each member of the couple must own and sustain their *voice* in the relationship. That is why so many come into therapy espousing the need to fix their communication skills. Effective communication is a hallmark of successful relationships. Harville Hendrix's Couples Dialogue Exercises are a mainstay in our work.[47]

Conflict is inevitable in life and certainly in passionate relationships. Possessing *conflict resolution skills* and effectively executing them to promote "win/win" outcomes is a critical couple's skill. Paul Shaffer, a colleague in North

Carolina, provides an excellent book and skills to repair lost negotiation qualities.[48] *Intimacy* is another vital component in a relationship. It is both the ability and the choice to be close, loving, vulnerable, and trustworthy. These components are important in supporting a couple: voice, conflict resolution skills, and intimacy.

The "romance love" that snares a couple into strong levels of attraction, lusty nights, intense sense of togetherness, and complete loss for the reality of time often fades after three to six months when the reality of life begins to intrude. Committing to demonstrate your love and respect for your partner through ongoing *romance* is one way to maximize the passion. How do you define romance? Romance demands that you think, plan, compromise, change, and mature. It requires that you give up the hope of finding the perfect partner and turn your attention to the task of loving and honoring your real-life mate. Women in couples' therapy often remark, "Having a romantic partner is more important than having mind-blowing orgasms or an expert in communication." So how do you create ongoing romance in relationships?

Three cardinal rules of romance are seeing the world through your partner's eyes, creating everyday excitement, and showing physical affection. Seeing the world through your partner's eyes requires that you discover what makes him feel "loved" by you. Does he feel loved when you send cards, write notes in his day planner, prepare his favorite meal, plan an evening away, dress up in sexy lingerie, and seduce him? The tricky part is that most people give what they want to receive, so be careful that you are not creating quality time experiences when hot sex is the ticket. Gary Chapman's *The Five Love Languages* is a great exercise to uncover how one wants to be loved. I totally agree with Dr. Chapman that love is a "verb," not a "noun." Love requires action on the part of a lover, and knowing how your partner wants to be loved is a sure way to his heart. If you have not uncovered how you wish to be loved, take the time for this fabulous exercise. His book is an easy read.[49] After yours are uncovered, ask your partner to join you and discover how he rates his.

Gary Chapman's Five Love Languages
- Quality time
- Physical touch
- Words of affirmation
- Acts of service
- Gifts

A true romantic invests excitement in the everyday, not just in great vacations. Do you surprise your partner with a waiting hot bath, a midnight picnic on an early spring night, or brownies for no reason at all? When relationships become predictable and routine, romancing the everyday is a sure solution.

Then again, planning a weekend away and never leaving the room is not a bad option, either.

Physical affection is an integral part of romance. Kissing, holding hands, sitting close on the sofa, snuggling, and loving massage are ways we reinforce the physical bond with each other. What type of physical affection does your partner appreciate? Role modeling physical affection for children of all ages plants the seed of romance, providing them with a template for their future choices in partners.

Nine out of 10 women who enter couples therapy tell me, "I could be more passionate and more in touch with my sexuality if I knew that every time I kissed him, cuddled a few minutes longer than usual, and sexually teased him he did not expect the affection to end in intercourse." Teaching partners to anticipate less with affection and enjoy the moment without dashing off to the bedroom has been monumental for dozens of couples. For a two-week period, I often put the partner overengaged with the physical in the role of saying no to intercourse. When they see their partners suddenly initiating touch, being seductive, and flirty, new possibilities form.

Romance does not have to cost a fortune, take a massive amount of time, or even tax your creativity. Laura Corn's book *101 Nights of Great Romance* and books like it are on the bookshelf in the bookstore.[50] Find one that is comfortable for you and commit to one romance deposit a week.

Romance Tips
- Make a daily effort to please
- Be mindful of anniversaries, birthdays, and possibilities for connection
- Involve the element of surprise—breakfast in bed, notes, or flowers
- Do something that costs nothing more than time—water the plants or wash the car
- Show mutual respect—don't interrupt, use eye contact, or turn off the television
- Be playful and flirtatious
- Be sensitive—write a poem or a love note or create rituals

THE PROMISE OF INTIMACY

People often enter midlife wondering what happened to the quality of the intimate connection they shared. It isn't that intimacy is lost to these couples; rather, it has diminished in quality. Emotional intimacy and physical intimacy are the two main parts of a romantic relationship. Problems with communication and intimacy are often cited for the reason people enter couples therapy. They are describing the need for emotional intimacy: closeness, sharing, and self-disclosure. However, when intimacy is the desired element for relationship renewal, they generally are asking for more sex or physical intimacy.

I see intimacy as a broad term to describe the many facets it incorporates. If intimacy is an umbrella term, then the spines of the umbrella that give it strength are expressiveness, compatibility, cohesion, sexuality, autonomy, conflict resolution, identity, and affection. Dr. Edward Waring developed a model for intimacy in the late 1980s.[51] It has been helpful to create talking points for couples to enlarge their view of intimacy and to assess the level of development for intimacy in the relationship. I have included an exercise in Appendix C. Circle the level of development (1–5, where 1 = low and 5 = high) you have obtained as a couple for each of the eight factors of intimacy; have your partner do the same. Discuss your results. Are they similar? Do you see patterns? The exercise opens a dialogue to enhance intimacy in your relationship.

Janet Woititz, in her book *Struggle for Intimacy,* writes, "Intimacy means that you have a love relationship with another person where you offer, and are offered, validation, understanding, and a sense of being valued intellectually, emotionally and physically."[52] Thus, intimacy gives you the freedom to be you. You are not judged; you do not have to walk on eggshells. You do not worry about making a mistake, and you afford your partner the same freedom. I find her description to be the most expansive to describe the qualities necessary for intimacy. Within the intimate bonds of a relationship, you celebrate your partner's values, interests, and separateness instead of looking for fusion or enmeshment. Your differences are either ignored or worked through.

At the heart of intimacy are vulnerability and self-disclosure. It is the process of verbally revealing the private self to another person through expressions of emotion, need, thought, and self-awareness. Is it any wonder that individuals have difficulty with developing and sustaining this link? How can you offer intimacy to another if you are unfamiliar with the inner you? Comfort with your inner self means that you can stand up for yourself in an intimate relationship without taking over the other person or losing yourself to the other. Relationship boundaries are acknowledged and maintained. Dr. John Bowlby, renowned attachment theorist and psychiatrist, offers another advantage to sustaining intimacy in relationships: "The quality and the quantity of intimacy in a marriage constitute the single most important factor of marital satisfaction and family function."[53]

A NEW VIEW OF SEXUAL DESIRE

Libido, lust, passion, horny, sexual interest, hot and bothered—there so many descriptors for *sexual desire,* and still the confusion remains. I believe that confusion about desire exists mainly because men and women are hard-wired differently. Men are indeed from Mars and women from Venus. A man's desire to be sexual with his woman can be easily ignited by looking at her body as she dresses for work in the morning. I do not intend to fault a man for this easy access to desire. My intent is to demonstrate the difference in our natures. Understanding the differences and moving toward acceptance of differences takes a couple out of the tug-of-war and onto solid ground for a prosperous future. A woman's desire for a sexual encounter with her man, especially if the menopause transition and changing hormones are embedded in her hardwiring, is generally not ignited by a view, a thought, a single kiss, or a casual touch. Sexual desire for women is more complex, a weaving of multi-colored threads into her fabric of life. The multiple roles she juggles make up her tapestry of life. Sexuality is merely one colorful thread in the tapestry. How bright the color and how pronounced the integration into the tapestry depends on her comfort with being sexual, how she prioritizes sex for their relationship, and how many other threads of life compete for her attention. For example, Lexie and her initial tapestry of life and integration of sexuality appeared void of sex. The color was a light pink, and it appeared only episodi-cally in the tapestry. Now, after her courageous exploration and Ben's support and patience, the color is a bright purple that is richly woven in a multitude of places with intensity and purpose.

How is sexuality woven into your tapestry of life? What color is it? Dis-covering ways to reinvest in sexuality through thoughts, energizing arousal, exercises to reveal sexual possibilities, and making the sexual enhancement of your tapestry a priority, whether you are with a partner or not, is sexual revital-ization for today's seasoned woman.

To become more enlightened regarding a woman's sexual desire and strate-gies to activate it, one can benefit from understanding the body's physical buildup and changes during sex. In the 1960s, sex researchers Masters and Johnson developed a linear process of *sexual response* with four separate phases: excitement, plateau, orgasm, and resolution.[54] Later, Helen Singer Kaplan re-vised the process of human sexual response, acknowledging that a woman's mind is a critical component for her sexual satisfaction.[55] The past two de-cades of research into women's sexual function by Dr. Rosemary Basson and others questions the linear view with desire as an initial awareness for women. Instead, researchers contend that the sexual response in women is more of a circular model with overlapping phases of response and that desire is triggered later in the arousal process, not at the onset.

Masters and Johnson's physiological picture of arousal and orgasm with the four phases are as follows:

Excitement: Men and women experience that the heart rate and breathing become more rapid and that the nipples become erect. While for women the vagina begins to lubricate and the outer third becomes engorged with blood, the labia and clitoris also begin to expand with blood, and a warm tingling sensation is felt in the genitals. Men find that their penis becomes erect and that the scrotum thickens while the sac elevates.

Plateau: Both men and women can find that their initial arousal builds with an increase in muscle tension, involuntary muscle contractions, heart rate, and breathing and that a sexual flushing on the chest, face, and breast begins to appear. Women may feel the tingling increase to a sense of fullness or even throbbing in the entire genital area; lubrication increases, the orgasmic platform in the outer third of the vagina becomes larger, and the inner two-thirds of the vagina expands to accommodate the enlarged penis, while the uterus elevates for more comfortable thrusting of the penis. The penis becomes fuller and the head a deeper color as it engorges with blood. Preparation for ejaculation is taking place as the prostate and seminal vesicles contract. Early seepage from the penis can occur that contains sperm. Ejaculation propels approximately 300 million sperm into the vagina, and it takes only one sperm to create a baby.

Couples wanting to savor the arousal and plateau process learn to stop and start the intensity of arousal without peaking too soon. A man's *point of inevitability* is the point in his level of excitement where he has reached threshold and will ejaculate. This choreography of lovemaking requires connection to sensations, attention to a partner's level of arousal, and often verbalized needs for additional stimulation to provoke the next phase: orgasm. Research has shown that with active thrusting, a man will often climax in less than two minutes, while it may take a woman much longer to reach orgasm; thus, the choreography of lovemaking can become an art of attending to each other.

Orgasm/climax: At the peak of sexual excitement, both experience intense muscle contractions, feelings of pleasure, loss of voluntary muscle control, and sexual release. Women note contractions in the vagina, pubococcygeal muscles, rectal sphincter, uterus, and clitoris and a series of spasms, depending on the intensity of the orgasm. Men note spasms during ejaculation and contractions of the prostate, testes, urethra, and sphincter muscle of the bladder to prevent sperm from being expelled into the bladder. The intensity of orgasms often varies, depending on the individual partner's focus and lovemaking intent. Women can experience multiple orgasms and some a gushing of secretions almost like an ejaculation; this is normal.

Resolution: The intense release after orgasm returns the heart rate, blood pressure, body temperature, and breathing back to normal. Relief of vasocongestion (pooling of blood) and enlargement of the breasts, genitals, penis, scrotum, and testes occurs as the muscles relax. Men have a refractory period or time of recuperation after orgasm that can take a few minutes in his twenties to a few hours or days with aging. Women do not go into a refractory period, allowing for multiple orgasms and a longer period of fulfillment.

Figure 8.3
Four Phases of Arousal

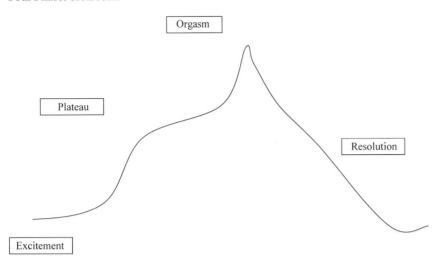

This "afterglow" period offers a couple time to experience the lovemaking connection and not necessarily run to clean up (see Figure 8.3).

Study into women's sexual response validates the initial findings of Dr. Helen Singer Kaplan that a woman's mind-set is central to her response and the further investigation by researchers like Dr. Rosemary Basson regarding over-lapping phases of response that are integrated into the mind and body of a woman. Several key features of the new model have been eye opening for in-dividual women and couples in sex therapy. The First is the acknowledgment that a woman's "desire" to be sexual at the onset is often neutral; however, with motivation, a willingness to receive and respond to sexual stimulus, and feel-ing heightened senses of arousal, desire can be ignited and a satisfying sexual encounter experienced. In sessions, I take women or couples through Masters and Johnson's linear process and then explore the new model by Basson.[56] Women, often for the first time, explore the concept of their sexual motivation or interest in being sexual. I have heard a variety of reasons and listed them for you to explore. Why do you initiate sexual activity or agree to sex?

Motivation or Interest in Sexual Activity

- To receive or share physical pleasure
- To please a partner
- To feel emotionally closer
- To increase her sense of well-being (to feel attractive, appreciated, loved, or desired)
- To relieve sexual tension

- Out of duty or guilt (it has been too long between sexual encounters)
- To escape punishment

Ideally, the *interest* and *motivation* come from a healthy view of sex and your relationship to your partner, thus leading to enjoyment and sharing of pleasure. I get very concerned when women proclaim, "I just 'give it up'; then I won't have to see him pout," or say so to escape the verbal punishment and withdrawal. Saying no to sex is a healthy decision to make versus having sex out of duty or guilt, or to escape punishment. Refraining from sex because of a lack of interest, tiredness, or physical problems (yours or your partner's) or because there is no current partner are all reasonable. Sex needs to be a free, pleasurable experience for both parties. Later, I discuss "maybe" opportunities for lovemaking.

The second phase in the process we discuss is *willingness*. Willingness to receive pleasurable stimulus via kisses, touch, and other stimulation and willingness to respond to the stimulation are critical aspects of this next phase. All too often, a woman may find herself agreeing to sex, only to find that the willingness "to respond" to touch is absent. You are the only one in the room in charge of this essential element. Gently push aside the interrupting thoughts regarding the dishes in the sink, the report that is due tomorrow, or the phone calls you still have to make and *focus* on pleasure and the positive feelings you have for the person wanting to pleasure you. Relaxation exercises and learning how to tap into the relaxation response and silence those interrupting thoughts may be necessary for your expertise with the concept of willingness.

The third phase intensifying arousal can require mastery in exploring and harnessing your sensual self. Arousal often requires a focus on pleasurable stimulation, positive feeling about your partner, and tapping into your senses. The Treasure Hunt Exercise becomes remedial work for many postmenopausal women. How does the touch excite you? Do you hear your name called, sensual music playing, or even guttural moans of delight? Has the candle evoked a thrill, or is it the cologne? Now, I have your attention. Imagine your ability to create a wicked level of response by igniting all five senses during lovemaking. It may take some imagination, intention, and practice, but I guarantee it is well worth the effort. We cannot expect the lusty passion of our early years to carry us through the hormonal decline—being intentional is a much better investment.

You have chosen to be sexual with your partner, your willingness to touch and be touched is engaged, your sensual self has ignited your arousal, and ultimately "sexual desire" has been triggered. You "want to be wanted," and the mind and body are responsive. This is a very different picture than the linear model, which assumed that desire was present at the onset of sex. And now, just a few words about the overlapping phases and how this circular process for women can be "short-circuited." When a woman lets interfering thoughts enter the cycle and focuses on them, begins to think about the element of "time," or remembers her partner's most unpleasant characteristics, a partner climaxes or loses touch with your level of arousal; if any or some of these occur, the sexual response cycle can be disrupted. The element of time can be a frequent culprit. He is giving her oral sex; she enjoys it at first and then begins to think how much time it is taking. Now her level of response toward orgasm has a long way to go, and the process is short-circuited. An option is to return to the senses, reengage them, squeeze the pubococcygeal muscles, and let the muscle tension grow; soon your excitement will return, and time becomes a nonissue.

In the fourth phase, you have mobilized your interest, willingness, arousal, and desire, and now the gift of sexual release—orgasm—is on you. Enjoy the connection with your partner with or without orgasm, the experience of afterglow, and all opportunities for a satisfying sexual coupling. Take the three to five minutes or even an hour to regroup and affirm loving feelings you share rather than jumping out of bed to clean up and casually talking together (see Figure 8.4).

Figure 8.4
Modification of Basson's Work

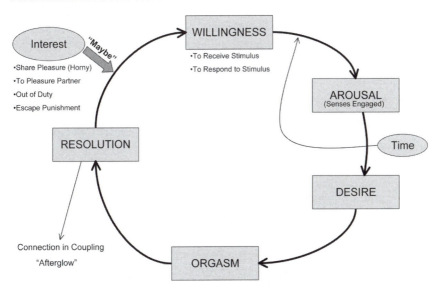

Source: "Woman's Sexual Dysfunction: Revised and Expanded Definitions." Reprinted from, CMAJ May 10, 2005; 172(10), Pages 1327–1333 by permission of the publisher. © 2005 Canadian Medical Association.

Spontaneous or initial desire does not set the stage for a woman's sexual response process. To further understand this evolving spectrum for desire, S. Michael Plaut's work suggests that an individual's interest in being sexual is determined by the interaction of three related but separate components: biological, motivational, and cognitive.[57] The *biological* impact of desire can be influenced by hormones, medications, illness, and other aspects that can physiologically impair the circuitry for desire. That includes genital stimulation, activation of the senses, or anything that slows down the arousal process. *Motivation,* the most complex but most elusive component, is particularly important for women. It involves the interest, psychological and interpersonal drives, emotions, and willingness to receive and respond to stimuli as explored in the earlier model. *Cognitive* factors are the thinking part of desire, such as beliefs, values, expectations about the sexual activity or relationship, and the need for satisfaction. The three components can be so interwoven that any one or all three cripple sexual desire.

On a positive note, let's attempt to use this information to a woman's advantage. A woman in the throes of menopause can benefit from all advantages— thinking or feeling domains. A recent woman in my office was disconnected from desire on many fronts. Linda is a 63-year-old married woman, a busy executive with three grown children and a loving husband. She enjoys her new freedom to come and go without the pressure of making dinner, driving children about, or even having to entertain Bill, her husband. They have great sex on vacations; the issue lies more with the everyday sexual connections. Minimal underlying relationship issues are present, they love and respect each other, and her hormones are augmented with a combipatch that she has used for three years after significant insomnia, flashing, and weight gain. Linda remarks, "You will have to hold me at gunpoint to take away my hormone patch. I feel more like myself than the three years I struggled without it."

Innervating Linda's desire in the three domains began with the biological process. To increase her sexual drive, she read erotic novels filled with steamy passages, considered how Bill would do the same things to her body, and even read excerpts to him at night as they lay in bed. This seduction prompted a sexual simmering and a tingling in her genitals. Next, cognitions or thoughts were energized. Linda values her sexual encounters with Bill. Her belief system includes sex as sharing, a passionate closeness, and a personal expectation to tap into her senses and release her own passion. Finally, her motivation to act or not act integrates her own need for sexual stimulation, the joy in watching Bill pleasured, and the fabulous connection they both feel when they do make love.

How can you maximize this composite of desire to fuel your momentum? If all three domains are engaged to a mild level, there is a 20 percent chance of a spark. If all are engaged to a moderate level, you have approximately a 50 to 60 percent chance of moving to sexual activity. When all are stimulated to a high level, systems are a "go"—just choose your activity.

SINGLE AT MIDLIFE

What if midlife finds you without a partner? For the seasoned siren that lies inside you, it may mean adjusting expectations, refueling the fires of passion, and celebrating new life. I am not suggesting that you go in search of a replacement. I am suggesting this is a time to journey inside—to make peace with loss and longing and open those spaces to life and love. It may be the first time you can really learn to love and appreciate yourself. There are women at this junction who have never lived alone; they went from their parents' home directly to the marital home and then into years of pleasing and performing for others. Now freedom to "be" awaits them.

Gail Sheehy describes the Pilot Light Lover as a transitional figure to re-ignite passion and sex for this new traveler in the world of lust. He may be interesting, successful, fun loving, a great lover, and even married (a minor detail left out in those early introductions). Pilot Light Lovers have a distinct purpose to recharge the battery, but they rarely last.[58] Enjoy the time you share, be honest with yourself, and certainly not desperate for love, or he will run for the hills. The problem often is that the midlife woman lets too much of her heart get involved in the seduction. Then bits and pieces need months to collect.

And then there are the stories of the 25-year marriages hit broadside by a midlife crisis, leaving a woman stunned but not down for the count. She reenters life with a determination to be her best self, not needing a man, but perhaps a companion for dinners, the movies, and concerts. Then another hit broadside occurs when Mr. Wonderful enters her life. This unassuming woman finds herself sleeping less, not stopping to eat, discovering intense energy, and losing weight without even trying. New clothes, business, and friends may find themselves on the back burner as she engages "new love." Hours are spent talking on the phone with a man she describes as "so easy to be with, it is as if we have known each other for years." And the joy of unbridled passion leaves her in bed for hours on the weekend versus her previous Saturday night routine with movies and popcorn.

The fantasy of a "boy toy" is another story for these divas. Some say that a younger man enjoys a woman for herself, her accomplishments, and her ability to talk about anything and that they do not have to worry about pregnancy. She doesn't need a man; she is fine on her own, and what he has learned from her is invaluable even if the relationship ends. Diane Keaton has done much to propel the image of the successful seasoned woman entering life with a new lover. *Something's Got to Give* with Jack Nicholson and Keanu Reeves kept me amused for days.

There are a few words of caution for single midlife women exploring passion. If you are perimenopausal and having periodic menstrual cycles, you could still be producing eggs and possibly become pregnant. Some form of birth control is a wise decision, so talk to your health care provider. What about safe sex for this population of lovers? Condoms fit as easily in a woman's purse as in a man's wallet. You have given "the safe-sex talk" to your children, so take your own advice and be cautious. Sexually active postmenopausal women with genital atrophy may be at increased risk for sexually transmitted infections (STIs) because of the vulnerable tissue in the vaginal that has thinned because of hormone changes. Women are twice as likely as men to contract gonorrhea, hepatitis B, and HIV if exposed. Symptoms may lie dormant, thus making it more difficult to diagnose and treat. Discussing sexual histories with new sex partners is responsible sexual behavior for all ages. Do not be embarrassed to ask a partner, especially a new partner who has been with multiple partners, to get tested for STIs and get tested yourself. Symptoms to have checked, even if they disappear after a while, are discharges, burning, itching, rashes, bumps, or sores that appear in the genitals. And do not forget those annual physical exams and Pap tests when necessary. Genital health is important throughout a lifetime, so why risk your health now? Besides, you are modeling healthy behaviors for the youth who follow.

STRATEGIES TO ENHANCE SEXUAL RELATIONSHIPS

This chapter highlighted numerous aspects of sexual well-being to assist the seasoned woman reinvent her sexual self. The following exercises demonstrate a variety of activities for self-discovery, a glimpse into the world of toys, lotions, and sensate focus exercises and how to create a sexual menu to perk up a humdrum sexual routine.

The first four exercises assist a woman in knowing her body and its parts and develop an overall comfort with touching. For some women, repeating these exercises, no matter how long ago you checked out your parts, creates a new relationship, especially when hormones may have altered your familiar pathways for touch. The knowledge you gain is better than any refresher course you have ever taken.

Body Image Exercise for the Mature Woman

Your body image is more than the physical mass you inhabit. To understand where you are now as the mature woman, you need to revisit your developmental years searching for themes, patterns, and the pathways chosen.

Set Aside 30 Minutes for This Exercise

Forage in your scrapbooks or photo albums or contact family members to send you pictures of yourself at age two, your school-age child (ages six to eight), the adolescent you (ages 12 to 16), the young woman (ages 18 to 21), the developing woman (ages 22 to 35), you in motherhood, the woman you became (ages 36 to 55), and the mature woman (age 56 to present).

Ask yourself the outlined questions for each era. What discoveries did you make?

Then proceed to the next session and make an appraisal of the many aspects of body image. Finally, jot a little note to the woman of today. How has she maneuvered through her journey? Do you have any tips for the future?

Questions for Each Era

What do you see in her face? What do you remember of the world she lived in? Did she have a joyful experience, or were there conflicts that had a negative impact? What discoveries do you have now regarding her evolving body image?

Body Image Appraisal

For each of the following categories, rate your comfort with the present level of development from 1 to 5 (1 = low level and 5 = high level). Make a note of your satisfaction.

Then note any changes you wish to make in that category.

[Example: Hair (#4) good length, keep it colored, no gray showing. No changes.]

Style of dress: (lingerie and outerwear)
Shoes:
Hair:
Makeup:
"The walk":
"Voice":
A note to the woman you are today: How has she maneuvered through her journey?
   Do you have any tips for the future?

Body Appreciation

This exercise, like a music appreciation class, enlightens your eye to the nuances of your body: the shape, size, and symmetry of all the parts gathered together for your unique appreciation.

Set Aside 30 Minutes for This Exercise

Enter the exercise with an eye for appreciation, not a critical review. Choose a time you are alone and will not be disturbed. Make sure the room is warm, try to use a full-length mirror for your investigation, and to enhance the experience play some music that is sultry and makes you feel good.

Step 1. Put on an outfit that speaks of your style of dress, something you enjoy wearing. Look at yourself in the mirror. Turn around and try to visualize yourself from all angles. Who do you see? Describe this woman in as much detail as possible. What do you admire?

Step 2. Now take off your clothes, slowly. Look again at the full-figured woman in the mirror. What do you appreciate? Shiny hair, a pert nose, a sumptuous mouth, pleasing arms, sexy hands, breasts that could tell a story, voluptuous hips, and sleek legs.

Step 3. What areas would you like to modify? Create a realistic plan and spend the next 90 days on your goal. [Example: Firm my buttocks, decrease the width by two inches over the next 90 days. Plan: Go to the gym three or four times a week, add buttocks exercises; measure at 30 and 60, days.]

Laura Berman's Genital Image Scale, Part I

Read the following items and check the category that applies to *your* feelings or thoughts about your genitals (i.e., labia, clitoris, vulva).

	Always	Often	Sometimes	Never
a. I feel anxiety and worry when I think about how my genitals function.				
b. I look at my genitals.				
c. I feel confident that I understand my sexual anatomy.				
d. When I think about my genitals, I feel ashamed or embarrassed.				
e. I feel comfortable/positive about my partner seeing my genitals.				
f. I have sad and depressed feelings when I think about my genitals.				
g. I feel ashamed/embarrassed about the size of my genitals.				
h. I feel ashamed/embarrassed about the shape of my genitals.				
i. I feel ashamed/embarrassed about the look of my genitals.				
j. I feel ashamed/embarrassed about the odor of my genitals.				
k. I feel my genitals work/function as they should.				

	Always	Often	Sometimes	Never
l. I am conscious of trying to hide my genitals from being seen by my partner.				
m. I feel my genitals are attractive and would arouse my partner.				
n. As a child/adolescent, I was self-conscious or embarrassed about my genitals.				
o. I use feminine hygiene products (douches, sprays, suppositories, and so on).				
p. Growing up, my family/caregivers gave me positive messages about my genitals.				
q. Growing up, I was given the message that touching my genitals was bad or dirty.				

Genital Image Scale, Part I: Scoring Template

Convert the following letters into numbers per question corresponding to scale:

Item Letter	Always	Often	Sometimes	Never
A	1	2	3	4
B	4	3	2	1
C	4	3	2	1
D	1	2	3	4
E	4	3	2	1
F	1	2	3	4
G	1	2	3	4
H	1	2	3	4
I	1	2	3	4
J	1	2	3	4
K	4	3	2	1
L	1	2	3	4
M	4	3	2	1
N	1	2	3	4
O	4	3	2	1

Item Letter	Always	Often	Sometimes	Never
P	4	3	2	1
Q	1	2	3	4

Part I: Range, 17 to 68

If you have a score of 17 to 30, you should consider looking at how your feelings about your genitals are impacting your life and sexual function. If you have a score of 31 to 68, it is on the higher end. You are in pretty good shape but should always look for areas of improvement.

Genital Image Scale, Part II

Check whether the following adjectives describe *your* feelings or thoughts about your genitals (i.e., labia, clitoris, vulva).

	Agree	Disagree

a. Unattractive

b. Embarrassing

c. Disgusting

d. Attractive

e. Malodorous (bad smelling)

f. Offensive

g. Inadequate

h. Healthy

i. Functional

j. Desirable

k. Well shaped

l. Good sized

Genital Image Scale, Part II: Scoring Template

Convert the following letters into numbers per question corresponding to scale:

Item Letter	Agree	Disagree
A	0	1
B	0	1
C	0	1
D	1	0
E	0	1

Item Letter	Agree	Disagree
F	0	1
G	0	1
H	1	0
I	1	0
J	1	0
K	1	0
L	1	0

Part II: Range, 0 to 12

If you have a score of 0 to 6, you should consider looking at how your feelings about your genitals are impacting your life and sexual function. If you have a score of 7 to 12, it is on the higher end. You are in pretty good shape but should always look for areas of improvement.[59]

Touch Yourself (Sensate Focus Touch) Exercise

It's finally time to get naked—always one of *my* favorite times. Carve out some private moments for yourself and head for the bedroom.[60]

The purpose of this exercise is to give your body a wake-up call and to reacclimate it to a new level of sensitivity. You're also going to track your body's reaction to touch. Here's the very simple way you're going to measure your body's response and level of arousal:

Level 1 = Zero to low level of arousal
Level 2 = Moderate level of arousal
Level 3 = Intense level of arousal
Level 4 = Orgasmic level of arousal

At each stage of this exercise, make a mental note of *which level of arousal you're experiencing.* Although you're likely to become aroused during the course of this exercise, orgasm is not the aim of the exercise. The aim of the exercise is to discover the wide range of response that exists between ice cold and orgasmic.

1. Lie down on your back. Take a few deep breaths. Relax. Feel the air touching your skin. Feel your heart beating. Close your eyes.

What level are you at?

2. Using your fingertips and starting at the very top of your head, slowly run your fingertips down either side of your head, keeping a light touch as your fingertips

stroke the length of your hair. Enjoy all the sensations that are created as you stroke your hair in this gentle fashion.

What level are you at?

3. Continue down your body. Begin stroking your neck and collarbone with the same gentle touch. Concentrate on feeling every nerve ending responding to the stimulation of your fingertips.

What level are you at?

4. From your collarbone, continue to your breasts and nipples. Go as slowly as you can. Feel the texture, temperature, and shape of your breasts and nipples. What is happening to your body?

   • Are your nipples becoming hard?
   • Is your rate of breathing changing?
   • Are you getting more aroused?

What level are you at?
Once you become acclimated to the stimulation and the intensity of the sensations begins to fade, continue down your body.

5. Stroke your sides and torso. Stroke your belly. Stroke your belly button. Ah, the belly button—a much overlooked, highly erogenous zone. Linger a little over that sexy, sunken little hole. Remember to keep it light and just use your fingertips.

What level are you at?

6. Now you're at the top of your pubic triangle. Lightly stroke your pubic hair. Slowly stroke the tops of your thighs and sides of your buttocks. Focus on the sensations your touch is creating.

What level are you at?

7. Lightly stroke your pubic hair. What does it feel like to stroke yourself so close to your vagina without touching it? Is it exciting to you? Part your legs. Lightly stroke the clitoral hood. Stroke the entire vulva (your external genitalia). Stroke the outer lips, the inner lips, above, below, and around. Remember that you're not *trying* to stimulate yourself with this exercise, although you most likely *will* become stimulated. See how aroused you become *without* having an orgasm.

What level are you at?

8. Although it may be hard to tear yourself away from ground zero, continue down your body, lightly stroking the tops and sides of your thighs and buttocks. Stroke your knees. Slide your feet toward your butt so that you can reach and stroke your calves, the top of your feet, and your toes. Take your time and continue to use a feather-light, fingertip touch.

What level are you at?
You have just stroked your body from head to toe. How do you feel? What level *are* you at now? Do you feel any of the following?

- A sense of well-being? (level 1)
- Warm and tingly? (level 2)
- Hot and bothered? (level 3)
- Explosively aroused? (level 4)

You may have felt all these various levels at different stages of the exercise. How does it feel to have completed the exercise? What is the lingering feeling?

Follow-Up to Exercise

Before your memory of the experience fades, look over the exercise again and take a minute to record your responses in a journal.

- What level of arousal were you at when you were stroking your head? Your neck? Your breasts?
- How long did it take at each station of your body before your arousal level started to climb?
- When is your arousal level the highest—when you first begin stroking your body or after some time stroking your body? Is the answer different for different parts of your body?

Knowledge is power. When you are intimately familiar with your body's responsiveness to focused touch stimulation, you have the power to quickly increase your own level of arousal. You also have valuable information at your fingertips that, when shared with your partner, will increase your level of pleasure and provide a powerful new avenue of connection with him.[61]

Kegel Exercises

Women have practiced Kegel exercises to strengthen the pelvic floor muscles after childbirth for more than 50 years. Dr. Arnold Kegel developed them in the 1950s to assist women with urinary incontinence. By contracting the pubococcygeal (PC) muscle, which connects from the pubic bone to the tailbone, women can strengthen the pelvic floor muscles, and the sexual response can be heightened, the vaginal opening tightened, and bladder and bowel incontinence reduced. Locating the PC muscles is quite easy. Practice by inserting a finger in your vagina and trying to squeeze down on the finger or by sitting on the toilet beginning to urinate and stopping the flow of urine by squeezing the muscles. Once you are familiar with the location of the PC muscles, strengthen them by consistent repetition. You can practice while on the computer, while on the telephone, or even driving in the car—the secret is consistency.

Tighten the PC muscles for a three-second count (one thousand one, one thousand two, one thousand three) as you inhale, then exhale, and relax. Repeat 10 times and then rest. Begin with five repetitions per day for five days, then increase to 10 times a day forever. This easy exercise has major benefits for your health and sexual satisfaction.

Scale of Relationship Intimacy

Intimacy is the glue that holds relationships together over time. How well developed is your level of intimacy in your relationship? This exercise helps you focus on the eight distinct factors of intimacy. For each of the factors, *circle* the level of development you believe your relationship has evolved into. Then discuss your reasoning with your partner. Chose one particular area to work on over the next 60 days.

You will find the Intimacy Scale in Appendix D.

Foreplay Revisited

Enjoyable lovemaking is not a linear process, that is, first a kiss, then touch the breast, then move to the genitals, and finally orgasm. If this has become the sexual routine, the next exercise can encourage both of you to take some risks and invite more pleasure into your lovemaking. Begin with the largest sex organ: the brain. Talk with your partner, tease throughout the day (a morning note on his mirror or a voice mail at lunch describing what you plan to do to his body at the end of the workday) and take your time approaching your sexual connection. When the normal pattern slips into the remark made by a recent client that "he touches my breasts, a few little kisses are placed strategically, then right to my clitoris," the satisfaction of *foreplay* is gone.

Remember how excited you got during young lovemaking? You touched and were touched and aroused to burning sensations in your panties—all with your clothes on. Men and women at midlife need to take more time to simmer lovemaking. The majority of women report that they need a minimum of 10 to 20 minutes to even launch enough arousal to begin lubrication or sensations to grow in their bodies. Carve out 10 minutes for revisiting foreplay and make sure your partner answers the questions, then share your results. Do you see any patterns or similarities? Over the next month, put at least three of your insights into action.

This exercise is meant to increase your awareness of your current style of foreplay and discover the minor adjustment that can propel foreplay into "hot monkey sex."

Rate each question from 1 to 4 (1 = never, 2 = occasionally, 3 = most of the time, and 4 = always), then discuss your answers with your partner.

I like to initiate sex with you.   _____

I want us both to initiate sex.   _____

I want you to begin the seduction early in the day.   _____

I want to cook dinner together before having sex.   _____

I enjoy going out to dinner and then having sex.   _____

Dancing with you is arousing before sex.   _____

Kissing passionately for several minutes is exciting.   _____

I want us to undress each other as part of lovemaking.   _____

I want to reserve an hour for lovemaking.   _____

Teasing me throughout the day simmers the excitement.   _____

Taking time to slowly touch all over our bodies is arousing.   _____

I like candles lit in the room.   _____

Bathing or showering together helps set the mood.   _____

Sexy music playing stimulates a sexy mood.   _____

I want to start foreplay outside the bedroom.   _____

Having sex in other places excites me.   _____

I get turned on telling you what I want you to do to me.   _____

I want to make love without going to intercourse.   _____

I enjoy a body massage as part of lovemaking.   _____

Watching erotic videos is arousing.   _____

I want to share my fantasy with you.   _____

I want to act out my fantasy with you.   _____

I prefer taking turns pleasuring each other for 10 minutes before sex.   _____

Reading erotic novels arouses me.   _____

Maybe versus the Automatic No

Because women often have objectives in mind other than sex, when a partner mentions a need to be together, this busy woman could respond with an automatic no. The Maybe Exercise brings a new option forth: "Okay, maybe I can warm up to the idea of sex—if the load of laundry gets folded, the report I was going to do tonight gets started, or I have a few minutes to myself to start my 'simmering processes.'" When the automatic no becomes common in the sexual relationship, resentments arise, and a rift ensues.

The Maybe Exercise buys you time to simmer. Simmering the idea for sex and considering your motivation to be with your partner is the first step. In addition, a woman tapping into fantasy, reading excerpts from her erotic novel, remembering previous loving encounters, or setting the scene that is arousing for you (candles, music, a bath together, or an evening walk on a warm night) moves her beyond the automatic response. Tell your partner that the idea is a "maybe"—you just have a few things to do first. Then set the simmering in motion, no matter how long you require, and keep your partner informed and then begin. For most people, once they begin a sexual encounter, after 10 to 20 minutes they are aroused and wanting to continue. The next step in a Maybe Exercise, is an understanding with your partner. You commit to trying; however, if after 20 minutes the arousal process is dull or absent, you either stop or re-negotiate another outcome versus intercourse. As I have said before, it is never okay to have intercourse if you feel the power of punishment. Share the Maybe Exercise with your partner; be sure to include the 20-minute clause and try it.

Basic Conditions Exercise for a Healthy Sexual Relationship

Good sex requires time, planning, and preparation. You cannot expect love to be the main ingredient. As with other parts of life, your sex life needs diversity. You would soon grow tired of watching the same movie or eating the same gourmet meal. So minor changes will augment an already good sexual relationship and help in the healing process for a relationship having difficulties.

The purpose of this exercise is to help you and your partner discuss, relate in detail, and attempt to meet each other's basic requirements for a strong and healthy sexual relationship. How sad that couples discuss their sexual wants at the onset of being lovers, but rarely do long-married couples reevaluate their sexual desire on the basics: time of day, lights on/off, or locations other than the bedroom. This exercise has become a favorite for couples as they attempt to release new sexual energy in their relationship. As you proceed with the exercise, keep in mind that most people have preconditions for sex that must be met for them to spark the intensity of arousal. What are your preconditions? Does your partner have a few? When was the last time you discussed them?

1. Make a list of the components that increase your sexual pleasure and comfort with your partner. Be as specific as possible. Include the following areas:

   Time: Morning, noon, nighttime
   Location: Bedroom only, anywhere, outdoors, public places, christen new places in the house
   Sound: Music, talking first, no talking, sexual sounds—moans, groans, "talk dirty to me"
   Lighting: Complete darkness, candlelight, soft lights, bright lights, a light from the distance
   Privacy: When the kids are asleep, when no one is around, not in other people's homes, not with parents here
   Mood: Playful, sexy, romantic, relaxed, not when upset, not stressed, sad, preoccupied, not with a fight

Sensory: Silk sheets, lingerie, costumes, using ice

Experiences: Exciting foods (whipped cream, honey, and so on), erotica, sexual vibrators, dildos, oils, powders, lubricants, toys

Accessories: Erotic literature, erotic movies, whips, bondage, anal toys, edible underwear

Fantasies: Bathe/shower together, pretend, act out fantasy, share a fantasy (couples should agree on a safe fantasy, and one should not feel pressured)

Process: Who initiates, how, how much planning, affection before, cuddling or talking before and after intercourse, afterglow—talk, hold, fall asleep together

2. Schedule uninterrupted time and share your list with your partner.

Are there preconditions that must be met for sex to be satisfying? Examples are hygiene, music, lighting, and no cigarette smell on the body. What do you *not* want to try?

Sexual Positions

Being creatures of habit, once you fall into a pattern of sexual activity, you tend to stick to that pattern. Think of the *sexual position* or positions you now use. When did you last attempt a new position? Different sexual positions can add sexual interest to your relationship, provide new stimulation, help with aging and the loss of flexibility, change the angle and depth of penetration, and afford you the opportunity for self-stimulation during intercourse and an ability to better stimulate your partner.

A word of caution. Have fun with the experimentation, and do not force a position. Take your time. If it becomes painful, stop and either try later or find another position. Allow for some mishaps and some laughter. The bottom line is that sex needs to be safe and fun for two consenting adults.

Lovemaking Styles

There is no better antidote to the pressure of living than a loving sex life—a sex life that has respect, variety, and fun at the heart. And there are times in our busy lives when a "quickie" is the preferred lovemaking style and then other times when we want leisurely touch and attention. I believe that most couples have a basic style and time period they devote to their lovemaking. I have created four types of lovemaking styles. Look at the styles and assign a percentage to each based on the number of times you and your partner engaged in them over the past year (be honest).

"The Quickie" is short and sharp and has a charm all its own. It allows a couple to take advantage of time, a critical resource we have little of these days.

You may have chosen a quickie when the children were napping (now it may be the napping grandchildren), before attending an appointment, or when the need to be sexual was immediate—"I want you, now."

"Amorous Awakenings" may creep in when you have less time than preferred and you want to be together. This style requires moderate time and energy. An example could be the early morning before work or your "tee time." Couples say that this gem can keep the sexual spirit alive all day long.

"Languid Lovemaking" screams for time, energy, passion, and a more leisurely pursuit of spirit. Couples returning from vacation recount the bliss of this style and the intense connections gained.

"Erotic Adventure" is about seduction, seduction, and seduction—those times when you yearned for the adventure and hoped you didn't get caught. Sex in the hammock outside, in the backseat of the car, on the beach, or even when christening the new furniture at home.

Treasure Hunt Exercise

Do you find yourself with less and less time?
Are the demands overpowering pleasurable moments in your life?
Does your passion appear silent?

Now is the time to revitalize your passion and pleasure. Tapping into your womanhood is a lifelong challenge. Do not let another day go by without discovering the *sensual* you. Your "sexual self" is the functional part of an individual that moves you to heightened levels of arousal and orgasm. But it is the discovery and reclaiming of the sensual self that ignites the sexual you to new levels of passion. Let the Treasure Hunt begin.

Whether you find yourself investigating passion for the first time, awakening pleasure silenced by the multitude of demands, or just affording yourself time to refuel, let this be a rich encounter. *Spend 20 to 30 minutes three times a week for the next month in discovery of your sensual spirit.* Alert each of your five senses for this revelation—what do you smell, hear, touch, see, and taste? You may choose to engage the senses walking in the cool morning air, watching a sunset, trying a new taste treat, reading a lusty novel, lingering over tea or coffee in the afternoon sun, or taking a leisurely bath. Just remember that this is a solo excursion.

- A warm bubble bath is an excellent venue for discovery. Collect items to enhance the excursion—scented soaps, loofah sponges, candles, music, a cool glass of juice or wine, or even bites of chocolate. Be sure to include a fresh towel and a robe or something pleasing to wear after your relaxing interlude.
- Now, begin to focus on your senses as never before. Sensual touch is not limited to a bath experience but is a good beginning for awakening passion.

- Candles, bath gel, and soap stimulate your sense of smell. So breathe in and out, slowly, as all the senses are heightened.
- Music can guide your mind away from those interrupting thoughts. Remember that now is not the time to plan the week's menu or solve work problems.
- Focus the majority of this experience on touch. What type of touch do you prefer: light, soft strokes with a washcloth; the tingling bristles on a body brush; or firm, circular motions of a sponge?
- I encourage you to begin with your face and slowly cover every part of your body with sensual touch, lingering at your breasts, genitals, and feet. Remember that you are on a treasure hunt. Let your touch awaken those sensual parts that have been dormant far too long.
- Don't forget your sense of sight. What do you see—bubbles, skin, fingers, and toes of a beautiful woman?
- Taste: what will it be? Sweet, sour, salty, or warm, cool, wet sensations—the choice is yours.

You have enjoyed a sensual trip. You "let go" of your worries and cares and delighted your body and senses. Now slowly, very slowly, rise from the tub. Wrap your body in a fresh towel, then gently smooth away the water drops from your body. One last sensation: cool lotion to moisturize your skin. Be sure not to rush this last moment of delight.

Remember the following:

- Commit to 20 to 30 minutes three times a week for one month.
- Take a slow, sensual visit with your senses.
- Focus on all the pleasures that surround you.
- Rediscover pleasure.

This could be a great warm-up exercise when you want to start the motor for sexual pleasure with your partner.

Over the years, women have enjoyed this so much that I created *Dona's Sensuality Bag for the Busy Woman* filled with all the items to delight the senses. It is available on my Web site at http://www.donasdelights.com.

Erogenous Awakenings

Erogenous zones are parts of the body that have a concentration of sensory nerve endings that, when stimulated, intensify arousal. These zones are divided into three levels of sensitivity. *Level 3* areas are less sexual in nature but create lingering sensations for delight. Massaging your partner's overall body with a concentration on the arms, shoulders, outer ears and earlobes, scalp, upper chest, buttocks, and calves will evoke the delight. *Level 2* areas have a greater concentration of nerve endings, producing arousal and sexual excitement. These are the parts you normally stimulate during foreplay: the back of the knees, inner thighs, armpits and breast, abdomen and navel, small of the back and buttocks, neck from back to front, the palms of the hands and bottom of the feet, the face (paying special attention to eyelids), edges of the nose, the temples, mouth, and tongue. *Level 1* areas are the most sensitive and sensual to touch: breasts and genitals. Great lovers explore the breasts and genitals with mystery, surprise, and teasing motions. Allowing the tension to build, then slowly pulling back while varying the stroking and technique, can move a passive partner into the land of bliss. Remember that level 1 areas should not be the immediate focus; vary the exploration in all three areas.

When was the last time you and your partner carved out time to explore these tempting areas? Because they can change over time as hormones and sensitivity to touch shifts, this is a wonderful opportunity for you to locate *three new erogenous zones on your partner.* Take 30 minutes for this exercise. Flip a coin to see who will be the recipient of the touch. Make sure the room is warm; a warm shower or bath is a good way to start. Now take some lotion, your partner, and your sense of exploration into a comfortable room and begin the adventure.

Sensate Focus Exercises

Sensate focus exercises were developed in the 1960s by Masters and Johnson to teach sensual touch and take the focus off of sexual performance and arousal. The goal is safe exploration and connection. Sensate focus 1 consists of touching and stroking the nonsexual parts of the body: the breasts and genitals are off limits. Sensate focus 2 adds breast and genital touch in an attempt to learn what pleases your partner. To receive maximum benefits from these exercises, I recommend you do each exercise two times over the next two weeks (set aside two one-hour times for sensate focus 1 and two one-hour times for sensate focus 2).

Sensate focus 1: The goal of this exercise is to be comfortable giving and receiving physical pleasure, not to produce excitement or orgasm. Carve out two 30-minute blocks of time during the same day. They can be back to back or after an hour or more of a break in which you switch roles. Flip a coin to see who the *receiver* will be. Ideally, the couple is to be naked for the exercise. The receiver lies face down. For this exercise the giver, is in charge of the experience. Select the room, music, lotion or oil, and other ambiances for the exercise. *The giver in not to touch breasts or genitals.* The focus is on touching, exploring the receiver's body, and discovering what the giver likes to do. Halfway through the exercise, the receiver turns over onto his or her back for additional touching.

The receiver is to focus on the giver's touch, noticing what is pleasurable, neutral, or unenjoyable. There is no communication during the exercise. At the conclusion of both massages, the couple will share their experience as giver and receiver. Even if sexual arousal occurs, no intercourse or an attempt at orgasm should occur during that 24-hour period.

Sensate focus 2: This is identical to sensate focus 1 with the addition of breast and genital touching to experience pleasure. The goal is not on performance or orgasm. In fact, even with the intense pleasure, the couple should restrain from intercourse and orgasm for a 24-hour period to maximize pleasure and anticipation of sex. Remember not to talk during the exercise. Share your experience, noting where the touch was pleasurable, neutral, or unpleasant.

To heighten the experience, try blindfolding each other during the receiving section. It can be thrilling not to know what to expect and where the touch will linger. You can also add sensory devices like feathers, ice, vibrators, and warming gel to spark the exercise.

Tantric Sex

Tantra was born in India more than 6,000 years ago, and today it flourishes in this country. Go to a bookstore, visit online book centers, attend a professional meeting, and you are bound to see a reference to tantric sex. My favorite book is still Dr. Judy Kuriansky's *Complete Idiot's Guide to Tantric Sex.*[62] Dr. Kuriansky's information is crisp and understandable, and the exercises help a couple venture into the land of tantra without being an expert. Tantra focuses on the deep connection of a couple to prolong the act of lovemaking, ways to weave together the polarities of male and female into a harmonious whole, opportunities to generate sexual energy, and rituals to promote bliss. I have indeed taken liberties and simplified tantra only to provoke your interest. Take the time to explore this ancient culture and bring new promise to your relationship.

Fantasy: A Normal Sexual Activity

Fantasies can be a mental image, a fleeting thought, or a deliberate mental wandering—they are normal. They occur in all people at any time of day. And since a sexual thought crosses your mind every 60 seconds, fantasy is just one of the fleeting thoughts that can ignite your pleasure. The 2004 AARP sexuality survey reports half of the 1,652 respondents state that they have sexual thoughts, fantasies, or erotic dreams at least once a week, with nearly one-fourth saying that they have those thoughts, fantasies, or erotic dreams at least once a day.[63] Fantasy can be anything from reading a sexy or erotic story to watching sexy videos to talking about things you would like to do (whether or not you actually go on to do it). Although clients I have worked with may say they feel shame or guilt and fear they are weird and try to suppress them, studies report that those who fantasize are in happy, loving, trusting relationships.

In fact, sharing a fantasy can be liberating and help couples feel closer, gain intimacy (self-disclosure is at the heart of intimacy), and accentuate arousal. If you have never broached the subject with your partner, first talk about fantasy in general and then ask what your partner's favorite fantasy has been or something he may want to try. Acting out a fantasy can be a rich addition to a sex life that has become routine.

One of my favorite resources is Laura Corn's *101 Nights of Great Sex*.[64] I often use this as an in-session consciousness-raising strategy. Her format is great. Each erotic encounter (once removed from the book, you have torn the perforations, which keep the content a secret) provides a list of ingredients you need for the encounter and a detailed script for your erotic experience. Couples commit to investing in the enhancement of their sexual relationship and surprise a partner with the encounter every other week. So consider a discussion with your partner, buying a book to help you envision fantasy and take the risk of acting out your sexual dream.

My research uncovered common fantasy themes for men and women: the Top Ten Female Sex Fantasies and Top Lesbian Fantasies. I have included them to spark your imagination and possibly open the discussion with your partner.

Cory Silverberg with www.About.com uncovered academic research articles on sexual fantasy—top sexual themes from the work of psychologist Harold Leitenberg and Kris Henning.[65]

Top Sexual Fantasy Themes

1. Having sex with your current partner
2. Having sex with a stranger or imaginary lover
3. Being forced or overpowered or overpowering someone
4. Group sex
5. Reliving a previous sexual encounter
6. Different sex positions or locations
7. Doing things you would never do in reality

www.AskMen.com reporter Vanessa Burton provides the following:[66]

Top 10 Female Sexual Fantasies

1. Oh, my virgin ears: Playing the innocent, naive, unknowing little girl who is taken advantage of
2. Strap me on, I'm going in: Dressing up like a man with a strap-on and dominating him
3. Two men at once: Being fawned over by two men
4. Leave a good tip: Being a stripper or prostitute

5. Three's company: Another woman to play with while a partner watches

6. Be her teacher: Have a master to obey, or not

7. Put her on display: Have an audience while engaging in sex

8. Who's your daddy?: Dominate a man: spank, order him to perform, and make him beg

9. The more the merrier: Group sex

10. Strangers in the night: Meet up with a mystery man and have a wild night of uninhibited sex

www.LesbianLife.com and reporter Kathy Belge offers the following:[67]

Top Lesbian Fantasies

1. One-night stands

2. Romantic

3. Delivery woman/mail carrier

4. Group sex/orgy

5. Celebrity sex

6. Exhibitionism

7. Dominance

8. Submission

9. Forbidden sex

10. Gender play

Developing Sexual Menus

Ponder the concept of a *sexual menu* for a few moments. Have your appetizers and side dishes become boring or nonexistent? Do you frequently move right to the main course, never considering a tasty little appetizer? Too many couples enter my office complaining of low sexual desire, lack of zest for sex, or the complaint that they need to spice up their sexual connection. Thus, the metaphor of the sexual menu was birthed, and it has electrified relationships once considered silent.

Here is your opportunity to develop your own menu. *Begin by carving out 30 minutes with your partner.* On a blank sheet of paper, brainstorm all the sexual activities you have shared over the past two months: kissing, showering together, necking while making dinner, oral sex, missionary position, rear-entry position, and time for afterglow. Using the following diagram, place each activity from your brainstorming in one of the following categories:

- *Appetizer*—Those comfortable actions that bring early excitement
- *Side dishes*—Activities that increase the passion, focus more on arousal
- *Main course*—Orgasm and intercourse

Your Sexual Menu

Appetizers	Side Dishes	Main Course
(Phase 1)	(Phase 2)	(Phase 3)

Taking time to create your menu and determining how excitement and increasing the arousal establishes new life to your sexual relationship is worth the critique. Do not be surprised when too few activities come to mind. By the second session, my clients have jumped into the process and begin to ask where fantasy and exploring erogenous zones belong. Is watching erotica in phase 2.5?

Vibrators, Toys, Lotions, Potions, and Paints

When were vibrators born? In the 1800s, hysteria, or womb disease as it was called, became the most common disorder among women. The symptoms were mental and emotional distress, a revolt by the womb against sexual deprivation. As many as three-quarters of all women had this disorder, and the treatment became doctor-administered genital massage that led to orgasm, or "hysterical paroxysm." Doctors and midwives were very busy until 1869; an American doctor invented a steam-powered mechanical device, the first vibrator. From steam powered, we have moved to the battery age and a diverse market for vibrators, dildos, and other novelties or marital aids. In the 1920s, the porn industry began using these "medical devices" in films, and an industry grew by leaps and bounds. It wasn't until 1952 that the American Psychiatric Association deleted the term "hysteria" from the diagnostic manuals. In 1994, an international symposium of sexuality scientists, the Fourteenth World Congress of Sexology, declared, "Sexual pleasure, including autoeroticism [masturbation], is a source of physical, psychological, intellectual, and spiritual well-being."[68]

Today's novelty industry includes sex toys, furniture, swings, real-life dolls, and more. This discussion is to desensitize women to the benefit of sex toys; they facilitate sexual pleasure. As long as toys are used consensually and pressure is not applied, these options to heighten pleasure are beneficial. I have been asked, "Isn't it weird to use sex toys?" My response, "Not at all." The 2004 AARP sexuality survey reported that after watching adult films together, use of sex toys was the second most frequently mentioned sex-related activity.[69] A University of California survey reported that 10 percent of American couples use sex toys in their sexual play.[70] Another common question in therapy is, "Won't the vibrator replace me"? That is doubtful. The vibrator produces an intense stimulation but does not take the place of a loving, compatible, supportive partner.

One homework exercise I have frequently prescribed for couples wanting to energize their relationship or for women breaking through sexual stall-outs is a visit to a well-run adult store. The other option is the multitude of online stores available; that offer reputable toys in discrete packaging. A list can be found in Appendix D. Two of the most popular toys are dildos and vibrators. Dildos generally are shaped like a penis without motors or vibration. Vibrators also have a penis shape but include a motor that can be battery operated or electrical. The Hitachi Magic Wand is the most well known vibrator with an electrical connection.

Several toys have gained popularity because of their design, action, and the pleasurable experience. Again, to desensitize and educate, let me share a few. The Pocket Rocket by Doc Johnson has remained popular since about 1995. This lipstick-size vibrator housing one AA battery is powerful but quiet. The Rabbit is widely known for its swirling shaft, undulating pearls inside the base, and external rabbit ears that flutter against the clitoris. The Rabbit received additional press when Charlotte in *Sex and the City* became addicted to hers, requiring an intervention from her friends.

Kama Sutra products offer affordable oils, creams, bath gels, balms, powders, and oil of love, most of which are edible. The Weekender Kit is a favorite of mine—a don't-leave-for-a-trip-without-it product that offers five different edible lotions to tantalize the weekend lover. But the Honey Dust is to die for. The lightest powder tasting of honey when applied to body parts in a temptress fashion can rock your man silly. Other products worth the investigation are edible body paints, chocolate sauce paint, blindfolds, restraint, or gently furry cuffs, Ben Wa balls, penis rings, bullets, vibrating eggs, anal dilators, nipple toys, and G-spot stimulators are others. An excellent resource to learn about toys, their use, and where to find them is *Em & Lo's Sex Toy: An A-Z Guide to Bedside Accessories.*[71]

A Few Words of Caution
- Read about the products materials, cleaning and care, and storage
- Have an understanding; if pain, fear, or safety are a concern, stop
- Always wash the item with soapy water and dry well before and after use
- If you are unsure what a toy is made of, use a condom on it
- Never put a toy that has been in the anus back into the vagina before washing
- Do not be lead to buy cheap products, as the quality is usually absent
- Store items properly to maintain their safety
- Keep spare batteries on hand
- Have fun and light laughter as you explore the world of toys

One last word on the world of toys toy parties. Have you ever attended one? Have you ever given one? Over the past decade, several companies have risen to the cry of the marketplace and now offer in-home parties selling products to promote intimacy and communication between couples. Passion Parties, Surprise Parties, Ann Summers, and Pure Romance are among the leaders in the market. Pure Romance is known in the sex therapy community for training their consultants to provide a safe and comfortable environment and knowing when to refer women to appropriate health care professionals.

Exploring Sex Video, Books, and Games

Adult videos, once regarded solely as a tool of erotic stimulation for men, have found a wider audience for couples seeking to heat up their sex lives. It is a safe way for couples to heighten passion and explore a wider range of sexuality. The new genre of *erotica* differs from traditional hard-core *pornography* in several ways:

- Sex acts are real and lustful, without a focus on ejaculation
- They have a real story
- There is a focus on sensuality and romance
- Women are featured as involved and equal participants, not objects
- They introduce a realm of erotic images and sounds into a couple's life

David Schnarch, Ph.D., says, "For many men, pornography is simply a way to experience sexual variety within a monogamous relationship. Men look at women in videos and magazines not just for their bodies, but for the promise that these women are highly charged sexually. And in this respect, older women have an advantage, women's potential to enjoy sex and to be an exciting, responsive lover tend to increase with age."[72] In other words, as long as a woman is willing and able to sexually satisfy her partner, the fantasy women of adult videos do not pose any threat. Even if a man or woman does, from time to time, rely on the explicit images of an erotic video to get "started," they can take that sexual energy and direct it toward a partner.

Erotica can also be a teaching tool for new techniques, positions, or a way to open sexual communication. In my office I often assign a couple a video, sometimes for education and also as a discovery for new levels of passion. *Becoming Orgasmic,* a DVD by Heiman and Lopiccolo, has moved anorgasmic young women beyond their lifelong barriers to orgasm.[73] The *Sinclair's Better Sex Video* series teaches couples sexual positions, oral sex, and advanced sex techniques, to name a few.[74] Candida Royalle's *Femme production,* videos made by women for women, are very well done and offer a naive woman new models for her budding sexuality.[75] In summary, sexual videos, whether educational or more erotic, are a positive intervention for a consenting couple.

Romance novels are a genre placing the emphasis on relationships and romantic love—a perfect equation for women stumbling through relationships with fleeting desire, fatigue, and little time for creative sexual outlets. My lending library to spark a woman's interest and creative imagery for their own sexual appetite supports the work of Sandra Brown, Nora Roberts, Kathleen

Woodiwiss, Lisa Kleypas, LaVyrle Spencer, and others. For some it may be the first time they have a book for sheer pleasure, and when they dog-ear a passage and share it with a partner in bed, the flames explode. The strong sexual content, sex scenes, and well-developed characters prove to be a winning combination.

I could not end this section without mentioning sexual games. A reticent couple introduced to a new board game, as a homework assignment, returns next week holding hands, exchanging glances and prepared for work. Some of my favorites are Romantic Rendezvous, Passion Game, Tantric Lovers Game, Kama Sutra, Speak Love—Make Love, and 52 Weeks of Naughty Nights. Games can be obtained online at http://www.simply4lovers.com, at the local adult store, and even Spencer's Gifts and Gags. Valentine's Day is probably a sellout opportunity for stores. So if you haven't tried one, make it a must-do.

The Kiss

A *kiss* represents an expression of affection, a show of respect, a greeting, a farewell, or our use of the kiss for sexual desire. The kiss has long been a global entity:

- History—The three types of Roman kisses
- Religion—The pope kissing the ground on arrival in a new country
- Folklore—Sleeping Beauty kissed to life again
- Art—Auguste Rodin's sculpture *The Kiss*
- Film—Lady and the Tramp eating spaghetti, leading to a kiss
- Theater—Romeo and Juliet
- Music—A long list, a favorite being Seal's "Kiss from a Rose"
- Photography—The kiss on V-J Day

Although the kiss is often lip based, nibbling with the lips on other body parts also has an appeal. Do you enjoy kissing your partner? Would you make any changes? Are you kissable? How do you know the other person wants a kiss? William Cane, author of *The Art of Kissing*, answers these questions and more.[76] Actually, clients discuss their dissatisfaction of their partner's kissing style frequently. Unfortunately, the answer to "Why haven't you discussed this with your partner?" is the retort "I did not want to hurt his feelings." So she pulls away from his kiss, stops the flow of passion after he moves to her lips, or chooses not to kiss at all because of smoker's breath or halitosis.

Kissing is more than an art form; it is another playful place for couples to share pleasure. If you have difficulties in the arena of kissing, move beyond the fear of hurting someone's feelings and in a caring voice, when he can hear you, tell him your concerns and get beyond the roadblock. I have collected 10 Kisses to Rock Your Partner's Socks, some of them are modifications from Laura Corn's *101 Nights of Great Romance* and others from years as a sex therapist.[77] Commit to one a week and see how the fun and excitement grows in your relationship.

10 Kisses To Rock Your Partner's Socks

- Surprise kiss—Say good-bye with a quick kiss; as your partner turns to leave, pull him back and place a passionate kiss on the lips.
- Phone kiss—During a phone conversation, take the phone away, tell the caller "Just a minute," pull your partner toward you, and give a passionate five-second kiss.
- Sweet kiss—Hold a sweet candy or fruit (strawberry) in your mouth, beckon your partner, and, while kissing, pass the fruit into his mouth.
- Don't you wish kiss—When your partner is with a friend, walk up, hold your partner's face, and place a kiss that stops any conversation.
- Ice cream kiss—Share an ice cream cone, lick it simultaneously; then, when mouths are cold, French kiss.
- Breakfast-in-bed kiss—Slip out of bed, prepare a "kissing breakfast" to serve in bed, pick foods that you can feed by hand, and kiss between bites.
- Emergency kiss—Kiss the palm of your partner; roll up the fingers, making a fist, then say, "Save this in case of an emergency!"
- Red-light kiss—The next time you are stopped at a red light, kiss your sweetie until someone honks the horn.
- Clandestine kiss—Tell your partner to meet you at a special place (closet, garden, or porch) at a specific time. On arrival, give your love a romantic kiss. Hint: Wear something fun like a trench coat, garter belt, or only a towel.
- Blindfold kiss—Whisper "I've got a little something for you" as you tie a blind-fold over the eyes; give a long, hot kiss on the back of the neck, a quick peck on the forehead, a longer kiss on the cheek, and one on the chin and shower your lover's face with kisses, leaving the lips for last.

My intention has been to fill you up with wild, bold, daring strategies that say "I want you, now!" The next step is for you to put them into the relationship on a consistent basis. Share a strategy you want to try or begin the seduction without warning. You are a seasoned siren committed to sexual revitalization.

Chapter Nine

ROMEO MEETS JULIET AT AGE 55

An archaeologist is the best husband a woman can have. The older she gets the more interested he is in her.

—Agatha Christie

Romeo had been divorced from his second wife for more than five years, and although he enjoyed the periodic visits from his 23-year-old son, this 61-year-old gentleman wanted companionship, someone to share life with. He met Juliet, age 55, on Match.com in the third month of his search. They discovered they had much in common from enjoying golf, walks on the beach, and movies to leisurely dinners. Juliet was new at the dating game, having recently been divorced a little more than a year from her husband Richard. Her friends had talked her into a membership on Match.com. Their enjoyment with on-line conversations became the evening's highlight—until Romeo suggested an exchange of phone numbers. It seemed to propel their relationship forward from the first vocal conversation. With an eagerness to meet face-to-face but a desire to be cautious, Juliet suggested coffee one afternoon. There seemed to be instant attraction for these two professional, midlife adults.

I met them some 10 months into the relationship. Juliet was referred by her gynecologist for perimenopausal symptoms and anxiety over a change in her sexual interest. Juliet had experienced early perimenopausal symptoms of irregular bleeding and periodic hot flashes for several years. During the first seven months of her relationship with Romeo, sexual attraction and desire was lusty, exciting, and very passionate. "How could things have changed? I still desire being with this man. I just do not feel like myself. And Romeo has noticed the difference. I told him it wasn't a loss of attraction; something inside me, the pilot light, was blown out!" she shared on that first office visit. Like so many women entering a provider's office, Juliet was confused by the changes in her body and her sexual appetite. She was a perfect candidate for some education into the world of menopause transition, the sexual response cycle for women (Basson's model), and some couples therapy to rewrite their sexual expectations and sexual menu, helping them both understand the chemical explosion of phenylethylamine hormones (PEA), the hormones of lust that are invigorating during the early month of passion but hormones that do not last forever. Then providing a menopause assessment and discussion of her options appeared to put them back into a loving mode instead of the anxious place they had resorted to. Juliet's decreased vaginal lubrication leading to some pain with intercourse was quickly resolved by an introduction to Astroglide, an excellent personal lubricant. She decided not to treat the hot flashes; instead, she made some dietary changes and increased her exercise plan. We have focused some attention on their sexual expectations in recent weeks and began the sexual menu to uncover what they do now and enjoy and what appetizers and side dishes they might want to add.

As new lovers in the menopause transition, they have several distinct challenges before them. What is Romeo's understanding of menopause and his previous experience with partners? What is Juliet's willingness to include him in her transition? What are their relationship strengths? Are there weaknesses to address? How compatible are they? What is their level of intimacy? What are their goals for the future as individuals and as a couple? Some of you may be able to identify with this list of challenges not as a new couple but from the perspective of sharing your life with a partner for many years and yet needing to readdress these relationship components to enhance your own relationship. This is another reason why many couples claim that the menopause transition offered their relationship new life.

SUPPORTIVE PARTNERING

Being a supportive partner during the menopause transition may require patience, putting your own issues aside for a short period of time, new enhanced "listening skills," and helping her as she makes choices for lifestyle changes or hormone therapy. Her success in the transition could depend on the quality of support she gets from her partner. Some women manage the transition with very little disruption in life; about 20 percent of women can coast through. A larger group about, 50 percent, experience mild to moderate disruption in life due to hot flashes, mood swings, sleep disruption, fatigue, and memory loss. Yet your partner may be in that 30 percent who have severe symptoms and will need hormone therapy during the process. It is important to note that menopause is as individualized as a thumbprint. Every woman's journey is different. Her needs are different, and her ability to share her transition with her partner is different. This natural process is not a medical condition.

UNDERSTANDING MENOPAUSE TRANSITION

A partner willing to listen, learn, and care enough to help his partner through the menopause transition is a gift during the process of change. Do you remember your mother going through menopause? Have you been through this process with another partner? Many men state that they were oblivious to their mother's transition. I asked my younger brother, Craig, who is now 47, if he remembered Mom in menopause. He didn't, and maybe that is a good thing since my memory is very vivid of her mood swings, her irrational state at times, and the relief when she had the hysterectomy. Sorry, Mom, but you were difficult during those days. I was 18 years old and probably not the most understanding (maybe even self-absorbed). I also remember my Dad on the golf course an inordinate amount of time.

An estimated 60 million American women are somewhere in the menopause transition or postmenopausal with an average of 6,000 women a day entering menopause. Women can enter perimenopause any time after age 35; the ovaries begin to reduce their output of estrogen. Menstrual periods become irregular and finally stop; the hormonal fluctuations can last anywhere from 1 to 15 years. As a woman approaches the final menstrual period, she may experience hot flashes and other symptoms. After 12 months without a menstrual cycle, she is in menopause and beginning her first year of postmenopause. Surgical intervention with hysterectomy, removal of ovaries, or chemotherapy and radiation therapy can induce menopause in women.

Common Symptoms Are the Following
- Hot flashes due to a decrease in estrogen
- Sleep disturbances, often from hot flashes or night sweats that interrupt sleep patterns
- Mood swings generally from a loss of sleep, an attempt to negotiate the various changes in her life from menopause, children leaving home, work conflicts, or unsupportive partners
- Vaginal dryness due to loss of estrogen that can result in a thinning of the walls of the vagina, loss of elasticity, decreased lubrication, and sometimes pain with intercourse
- Changes in sexual desire

Other effects on women during menopause are the risk for osteoporosis or weakening of the bones as estrogen decreases and the loss of elasticity of other body organs, such as the muscle tone of the bladder, causing women to lose urine when they sneeze, cough, or even laugh. Skin and breast changes are another part of the process, as estrogen is limited and the skin loses its durability. For a woman who has attempted to maintain her attractiveness and healthy body, the massive changes can be very difficult to deal with and may lead to sadness, depression, or even anxiety.

Six Essential Strategies for the Supportive Partner

1. *Adjust your attitude and expectations.* Understanding the physical causes of menopause and encouraging your partner to talk about what she is experiencing opens communication pathways and promotes understanding between a couple.

2. *Listen to her.* Do not try to fix it. This is a natural behavior for a man, but she doesn't need to be fixed. Rather, she needs to talk about what is going on with her body and have you listen and understand.

3. *Do not become defensive.* Her mood swings are generally not about you. What she may be experiencing is the sense that an "alien life force" is taking over her body. This is not the time to ask, "Did you take your medicine today?"

4. *Learn about the changes your partner is experiencing.* Knowledge is a powerful force. She will feel heard and understood when you ask how she is feeling, whether there is anything you can do, and when you share the knowledge you have unearthed about menopause. Hardly a week goes by without an article in the newspaper, on the news, or in *Men's Health* magazine and other periodicals.

5. *Support her lifestyle changes or hormone therapy.* Lifestyle changes such as exercise, diet, and stress management are often the first activities a health care provider will encourage. Weight gain is one of the most frustrating issues for women, as the weight seems to gather in the stomach and hips. One way of supporting her is to join in exercise or take up golf, walking, or biking. If these changes are not sufficient, your partner may find hormone therapy to be beneficial. A health care provider will discuss the risks and benefits before prescribing. Some options are dietary supplements, bioidentical hormone therapy, or other prescription hormones. Be part of the discussion and support her decisions.

6. *Help with tasks.* As estrogen declines, often a woman's endurance slips, she is easily fatigued, she may be getting less sleep because of hot flashes, or she may simply not feel like herself, thus making daily tasks at home or at work seem overwhelming. A supportive partner can help with the cleaning, cooking, shopping, or dishes— any help is so appreciated. The last thing your partner needs is to feel alone in this.

By being a supportive partner and attempting these six strategies, you could benefit greatly. A woman who feels valued and understood can move more easily to a loving, sexual place with her partner.

RELATIONSHIP ENHANCEMENT

This is a perfect time in the life of a relationship to take the pulse. Regardless of the length of time you have been together, it is never too early to reflect on your strengths, weaknesses, elements of compatibility, and levels of intimacy. Can you identify three *strengths* in your relationship? Strengths can be your ability to communicate, your listening skills, the conflict resolution abilities of the couple, and how you honor and respect one another.

What about those prickly parts of the relationship? Does she ignore your conversations about work? Do you feel that you have to beg for sex? When was the last time your partner initiated passionate love? Is money spent unwisely, or do you have a budget and pay bills together? The *weakness* in a relationship—those weak links—can unearth even the most committed relationship if they are avoided.

Compatibility is the ability of a couple to work and play well together. All too often, I meet couples who work together just fine; it is the playful part they have difficulty with. One of my favorite homework assignments in therapy is to send a couple home with the task of coming to a consensus on a playful activity and doing it before they return. Disconnected couples return without executing the homework—not because they do not know what is playful but because they avoid the intimacy of the discussion and putting play into action. How sad.

LEVEL OF INTIMACY

Emotional and physical intimacy are the two main parts of a romantic relationship. Emotional intimacy is described as the closeness, sharing, and self-disclosure in a relationship. Couples asking for intimacy to "renew a connection" are often talking about sex or physical intimacy. My belief is that intimacy is a broad term to express these two dimensions in a relationship. The eight factors that demonstrate a couple's level of intimacy are conflict resolution, affection, cohesion, sexuality, compatibility, identity, autonomy, and expressiveness. I invite you to visit Appendix C and review the Scale of Relationship Intimacy with your partner. Circle the level of development you have obtained as a couple in each of the areas. Then compare notes and focus on one or two of the areas over the next month. What can you do to enhance those two components? All couples can afford a little zest in their relationship; let this be your opportunity.

I challenge you in one more arena: the future. Use the intimacy factor of expressiveness and discuss with your partner your future goals as an individual and as a couple. When was the last time you ventured into the future in an intimate dialogue? Midlife begs the question, What does aging mean to you? Will you hit your stride or hit the wall? Retirement or reinventing yourself—in which avenue will you chart a course?

INSIGHT FROM THE PARTNER'S FOCUSED GROUP

I must thank the gentlemen who joined me to share their story as a partner of a menopausal woman. I began the evening asking what they remembered of their mother's transition and their overall view of menopause. Not one in the group could remember what Mom experienced. In fact, they did not harbor a particular view of menopause as either positive or negative. Now I am sorry I did not ask that question in the women's focused group. I imagine that the memories would have been different since a girl bears witness to her mother's journey and the role modeling that mothers do for their daughters. Next I asked them to review the typical symptoms that occur in peri- and post-menopause. These participants described vividly the course they traveled with a partner. It was interesting when asked which symptoms from the laundry list affected them most; the majority described weight gain, breast tenderness, change in sexual desire, loss of lubrication, and hot flashes. How interesting—sexual symptoms. They could not remember when symptoms started or how long they really lasted. Most of the women toughed it out and, according to their partners, did not have hormone therapy. Another interesting component of the focused group was when I asked what stories they wanted to share. I wasn't ready for the new cooling device one husband offered his wife during hot flashes: the CPAP hose from his face mask. Another participant felt that "warming gels" were a great invention.

What words of wisdom would you like to share with other partners or men in the future? "Be patient and understanding," "educate yourself about what is happening with your wife," "keep reminding yourself you do love her," "there is nothing to be afraid of," "time changes all things"—what a pleasure to be with a group of supportive men wanting to understand the process and be there for their woman.

APPENDIX A: COPING TECHNIQUES FOR TODAY'S BUSY WOMAN

Stress is inevitable. Positive coping skills will keep you resilient. Be cautious with negative coping skills such as alcohol, overeating, smoking, indulging, denial, and anger.

Identify your current coping skills with a circle and place a star next to two or three you want try.

Diversions

Get aways—time alone, movies, daydream

Hobbies—journal, write, paint, garden

Learning—take a class, read, join a club

Music—listen to music, play an instrument, sing

Play—goof off, play a game, go out with friends

Work—tackle a new project, keep busy, volunteer

Mental

Imagination—look for humor, dream, relaxation

Life planning—set clear goals, make a plan

Organize—make order, take charge, don't pile up

Problem solve—solve yourself, seek help

Relabel—change perspective, look for good

Time management—work smart, not hard

Relationship

Balance—time for work and leisure

Conflict resolution—look for win/win, forgive

Physical

Biofeedback—listen to your body, know limits

Exercise—walk, jog, swim, yoga, dance

Relationship (*continued*)

Esteem building—focus on personal strength

Flexibility—take on new roles, be open to change

Network—develop various relationships, resources

Togetherness—build traditions, express affection, take time

Interpersonal

Affirmation—say positive statements, believe it

Assertiveness—state your needs and wants, say no respectfully

Contact—really listen to others, make new friends, touch

Expression—show feelings, share feelings

Limits—drop some involvements, accept others boundaries

Link—share problems with others, ask for support

Physical (*continued*)

Nourishment—eat for health, limit use of alcohol

Relaxation—progressive muscle, breathe, warm bath

Self-care—take time, be reflective, energize the self

Stretching—take stretch breaks throughout the day

Spiritual

Commit—take up a worthy cause, invest yourself

Faith—find purpose and meaning, trust in higher power

Prayer—ask forgiveness, give thanks, gratitude, confess

Surrender—let go of problems, learn to live with situation

Value—set priorities, be consistent, spend time/energy wise

Worship—share beliefs with others, put faith in actions

APPENDIX B: NEGATIVE COPING SKILLS

Stress can undermine even the most resilient person. Negative coping skills provide an immediate relief for the stressed individual; however, they do not add to a healthy foundation.

Circle all the copers you currently use for stress relief.

Alcohol	Drink to change your mood. Use alcohol as a friend.
Denial	Pretend nothing is wrong. Lie. Ignore the problem.
Drugs	Abuse coffee, medications. Smoke pot.
Eating	Binge eating. Go on a diet. Use food to console.
Fault-Finding	Have a judgmental attitude. Complain. Criticize.
Illness	Develop headaches/nervous stomach/major illness. Become accident prone.
Indulging	Stay up late. Sleep in. Buy on impulse. Waste time.
Passivity	Hope it gets better. Procrastinate. Wait for a lucky break.
Revenge	Get even. Be sarcastic. Talk mean.
Stubbornness	Be rigid. Demand your way. Refuse to be wrong.
Tantrums	Yell. Mope. Pout. Swear. Drive recklessly.
Tobacco	Smoke to relive tension. Smoke to be "in."
Withdrawal	Avoid the situation. Skip work. Keep feelings to yourself.
Worrying	Fret over things. Imagine the worst.

APPENDIX C: SCALE OF RELATIONSHIP INTIMACY

Circle the level of development obtained by the couple in each of the areas in the following table. Then discuss with your partner.

Intimacy Factors	Beginning Level			Highest Level	
1. Conflict Resolution The ease with which differences of opinion are resolved	1	2	3	4	5
2. Affection The degree to which feelings of emotional closeness are expressed by the couple	1	2	3	4	5
3. Cohesion A feeling of commitment to the relationship	1	2	3	4	5
4. Sexuality a. The degree to which sexual needs are communicated	1	2	3	4	5
b. The degree to which sexual needs are fulfilled	1	2	3	4	5
5. Compatibility a. The degree to which the couple can work together and share tasks	1	2	3	4	5
b. The degree to which the couple can play together	1	2	3	4	5

Intimacy Factors	Beginning Level			Highest Level	
6. Identity Couple's level of self-confidence and self-esteem	1	2	3	4	5
7. Autonomy a. Success of couple to gain independence from family of origin	1	2	3	4	5
b. Success to gain independence from their offspring	1	2	3	4	5
8. Expressiveness The degree to which thoughts, beliefs, attitudes, and feelings are shared within the relationship	1	2	3	4	5

APPENDIX D: RESOURCE WEB SITES

Alzheimer's Association, www.alz.org.
American Association of Sexuality Educators, Counselors and Therapists, www.aasect.org.
American Cancer Society, www.cancer.org.
American Heart Association, www.americanheart.org.
International Academy of Compounding Pharmacies, www.iacprx.org.
Mayo Clinic, www.mayoclinic.com.
National Center for Complementary and Alternative Medicine, www.nccam.gov.
National Institute on Aging, www.nih.seniorhealth.
National Institute of Mental Health, www.nimh.gov.
National Osteoporosis Foundation, www.nof.org.
National Women's Health Information Center, www.4women.gov/menopause.
North American Menopause Society, www.menopause.org.
Sexuality Information and Education Council of the United States, www.siecus.org.

HORMONE TESTING

Diagnostechs, Inc., www.diagnostechs.com.
Genova Diagnostics (formerly Great Smokies Diagnostics), www.gdx.net.
ZRT Laboratory, www.zrtlab.com.

SEX THERAPISTS

Laura Berman, PhD, www.bermancenter.com.
Dona Caine-Francis, PMHCNS/NP-BC, www.magnificentmenopause.com.

SEXUAL AIDS

Eve's Garden, www.evesgarden.com.
Good Vibrations, www.goodvibes.com.

SEXUAL RETREATS

Sexplore Weekend Retreats for Couples.
Dona Caine-Francis, PMHCNS/NP-BC, www.magnificentmenopause.com.

NOTES

CHAPTER 1

1. Gail Sheehy, *The Silent Passage* (New York: Pocket Books, 1998), 27.

2. Lonnie Barbach, *The Pause* (New York: Plume Books, 1993).

3. North American Menopause Society, *Menopause Practice: A Clinician's Guide,* 3rd ed. (Cleveland: North American Menopause Society, 2007), 9.

4. Institute for the Future, *American Knowledge Workers across the Generations: Eight Dynamic Dimensions* (Menlo Park, CA: Institute for the Future), 2001.

5. Ibid.

6. Ibid.

7. Reynol Junco and Jeanna Mastrodicasa, *Connecting to the Net. Generation: What Higher Education Professionals Need to Know about Today's Students* (Washington, D.C.: National Association of Student Personnel Administrators, 2007).

8. Thomas Perls, "The New England Centenarian Study," Boston University School of Medicine, http://bumc.bu.edu/Dept/ContentPF.aspx?PageID=5749&DepartmentID=361 (accessed February 23, 2008).

9. "Centenarian," Wikipedia, http://en.wikipedia.org/wiki/Centenarian (accessed February 23, 2008).

10. Sheehy, *The Silent Passage,* p. 27.

11. Gail Sheehy, *Sex and the Seasoned Woman: Pursuing the Passionate Life* (New York: Random House, 2006), p. 50.

12. Ibid.

CHAPTER 2

1. North American Menopause Society, *Menopause Practice: A Clinician's Guide,* 3rd ed. (Cleveland: North American Menopause Society, 2007), 9.

2. Ibid., 58.

3. Gail Sheehy, *The Silent Passage* (New York: Pocket Books, 1998), 27.

4. Christiane Northrup, *The Wisdom of Menopause* (New York: Bantam Books, 2001), 106.

5. Robert Greene and Leah Feldon, *Perfect Balance* (New York: Three Rivers Press, 2005), 21.

6. Ibid., 12.

7. Eldred Taylor and Ava Bell-Taylor, *Are Your Hormones Making You Sick? A Woman's Guide to Better Health Through Hormonal Balance* (Atlanta: Physicians Natural Medicine, 2006), 17.

8. Ibid., 27.

CHAPTER 3

1. Gail Sheehy, *The Silent Passage* (New York: Pocket Books, 1998), 21.

2. North American Menopause Society, *Menopause Practice: A Clinician's Guide,* 3rd ed. (Cleveland: North American Menopause Society, 2007), 21.

3. Pat Wingert and B. Kantrowitz, "Is It Hot in Here? Or Is It Me?: The Complete Guide to Menopause," *Newsweek,* January 15, 2007, 38–54.

4. North American Menopause Society, *Menopause Practice,* 21.

5. Ibid.

6. Merrill Hayden, "Endometrial Ablation," *WebMD,* http://women.webmd.com/endometrial-ablation-1620 (accessed February 2, 2008).

7. "Hysterectomy," Wikipedia, http://www.wikepedia.org/wiki/hysterectomy (accessed February 2, 2008).

8. Hetal B. Gor, "Hysterectomy," emedicine, http://www.emedicine.com/med/topic 3315.htm (accessed February 2, 2008).

9. Ibid., p. 2.

10. North American Menopause Society, *Menopause Practice,* 21.

11. Ibid.

12. Ibid.

13. Robert Greene and Leah Feldon, *Perfect Balance* (New York: Three Rivers Press, 2005), 334.

14. North American Menopause Society, *Menopause Practice,* 21.

15. Ibid.

16. Health Body & Mind, "Hot Flashes? What to do right now," *Health,* October, 2007, 84.

17. L. Lindh-Astrand and E. Nedstrand, "Vasomotor Symptoms and Quality of Life in Previously Sedentary Postmenopausal Women Randomized to Physical Activity or Estrogen Therapy [in process citation]," *Maturitas* 48, no. 2 (2004): 97–105.

18. DermaTherapy (http://www.dermatherapyfabrics.com), Cool Sets (http://www.coolsets.com), and Wild Bleu (http://www.wildbleu.com).

19. North American Menopause Society, *Menopause Practice,* 21.

20. S. Bent and A Padula, "Valerian for Sleep: A Systematic Review and Meta Analysis," *American Journal of Medicine* 119 (2006): 1005–1012.

21. Barbara Swanson, "A Naturally Good Sleep," *Advance for Nurses* 12 (2007): 37.

22. North American Menopause Society, *Menopause Practice,* 21.

23. Ibid.

CHAPTER 4

1. Robert Greene and Leah Feldon, *Perfect Balance* (New York: Three Rivers Press, 2005), 4.

2. North American Menopause Society, *Menopause Practice: A Clinician's Guide,* 3rd ed. (Cleveland: North American Menopause Society, 2007), 858.

3. Alison Rigby and Jun Ma, "Women's Awareness and Knowledge of Hormone Therapy Post—Women's Health Initiative," *Menopause* 14, no. 5 (2007): 853–58.

4. Nurses' Health Study II, "The Nurses' Health Study Annual Newsletter," *Nurses' Health Study* 14 (2007), http://www.channing.harvard.edu/nhs/newsletter/index.html (accessed February 17, 2008).

5. Guttmacher Institute, "Multiple Factors, Including Genetic and Environmental Components, Influence When Menopause Begins," *Family Planning Perspectives,* 33, no. 5 (September/October 2001), http://www.guttmacher.org/pubs/journal/3323601.html (accessed February 17, 2008).

6. C. M. Farquhar and J. Marjoribanks, "Long Term Hormone Therapy for Perimenopausal and Postmenopausal Women," *Cochrane Database of Systematic Reviews,* Issue 3 (2005), http://www.cochrane.org/reviews/en/ab004143.html (accessed February 17, 2008).

7. Christiane Northrup, *The Wisdom of Menopause* (New York: Bantam Books, 2006), 169.

8. Ira Helenius and Deborah Korenstein, "Changing Use of Hormone Therapy among Minority Women since the Women's Health Initiative," *Menopause* 14 (March/April 2007): 2.

9. N. Smith and S. Heckbert, "Esterified Estrogens and Conjugated Equine Estrogens and the Risk of Venous Thrombosis," *Journal of the American Medical Association* 292: 1581–87.

10. Food and Drug Administration, "FDA Takes Action against Compounded Menopause Hormone Therapy Drugs," *FDA News,* January 9, 2008, http://www.fda.gov/bbs/topics/NEWS/2008/NEW01772.html (accessed February 17, 2008).

11. North American Menopause Society, *Menopause Practice,* p. 858.

12. American College of Obstetricians and Gynecologists, *No Scientific Evidence Supporting Effectiveness or Safety of Compounded Bioidentical Hormone Therapy,* October 31, 2005, http://www.acog.org/from_home/publications/press_releases/nr10-31-05-1.cfm (accessed February 17, 2008).

13. Harvard Health Publications, *BioIdentical Hormones: "Natural" Doesn't Necessarily Mean Better, Reports Harvard Women's Health Watch,* http://www.health.harvard.edu/press_releases/bioidentical-hormones.htm (accessed February 17, 2008).

14. North American Menopause Society, *Menopause Practice,* 858.

15. Ibid.

16. W. Somboonporn and S. Davis, "Testosterone for Peri- and Postmenopausal Women," *Cochrane Database of Systematic Reviews,* Issue 4 (2005), Article No. CD004509, http://www.cochrane.org/reviews/en/ab004509.html (accessed February 17, 2008).

17. S. Davis and S. Davidson, "Circulating Androgen Levels and Self-Reported Sexual Function in Women," *Journal of the American Medical Association* 294 (2005): 91–96.

CHAPTER 5

1. Chris Crowley and Henry Lodge, *Younger Next Year: Live Strong, Fit and Sexy-until You're 80 and Beyond* (New York: Workman Publishing, 2007).

2. U.S. Preventive Services Task Force, *Guide to Clinical Preventive Services* (Washington, D.C.: U.S. Department of Health and Human Services, 2005).

3. Michael Roizen and Mehmet Oz, *You Staying Young: The Owner's Manual for Extending Your Warranty* (New York: Free Press, 2007), 43.

4. P. Barnes and E. Powell-Griner, *CDC Advance Data Report #343. Complementary and Alternative Medicine Use among Adults: United States, 2002,* http://nccam.nih.gov/news/camstats.htm (accessed February 17, 2008).

5. American Heart Association, "Heart Disease and Stroke Statistics—2006 Update: A Report from the American Heart Association Statistics Committee and Stroke Statistics Committee," *Circulation* (2006): 113.

6. American Heart Association, *Metabolic Syndrome,* http://americanheart.org/presenter.jhtml?identifier=4756 (accessed February 25, 1008).

7. North American Menopause Society, *Menopause Practice: A Clinician's Guide,* 3rd ed. (Cleveland: North American Menopause Society, 2007), 137.

8. Robert Greene and Leah Feldon, *Perfect Balance* (New York: Three Rivers Press, 2005), 154.

9. North American Menopause Society, *Menopause Practice,* 137.

10. Ibid.

CHAPTER 6

1. Gail Sheehy, *Sex and the Seasoned Woman: Pursuing the Passionate Life* (New York: Random House, 2006).

2. Pia Melody, *Facing Codependence: What It Is, Where It Comes from, How It Sabotages Our Lives* (New York: HarperCollins, 1989).

3. Gail Sheehy, *Sex and the Seasoned Woman.*

4. Ibid.

5. Ibid.

6. Ibid.

7. Pat Wingert and Barbara Kantrowitz, *Is It Hot in Here? Or Is It Me?: The Complete Guide to Menopause* (New York: Workman, 2006), 203.

8. M. Keller, "A Comparison of Nefazodone, the Cognitive Behavioral Analysis System of Psychotherapy, and Their Combination for the Treatment of Chronic Depression," *New England Journal of Medicine* 342: 1462–70.

9. Wingert and Kantrowitz, *Is It Hot in Here? Or Is It Me?*

CHAPTER 7

1. Michael O'Shea, "How Stress Makes You Flabby," *Parade,* December 2, 2007, http://parade.com/articles/editions/2007/edition_12–02–2007/How_Stress_Makes_You_ (accessed February 25, 2008).

2. North American Menopause Society, *Menopause Practice: A Clinician's Guide,* 3rd ed. (Cleveland: North American Menopause Society, 2007), 259.

3. Yali Bair and Ellen Gold, "Ethnic Differences in Use of Complementary and Alternative Medicine at Midlife: Longitudinal Results from SWAN Participants," *American Journal of Public Health* 92, no. 11 (2002): 1832–40.

4. A. Vincent and D. Barton, "Acupuncture for Hot Flashes: A Randomized, Sham-Controlled Clinical Study," *Menopause* 14 (2007): 45–52.

5. "Mind/Body Medicine," http://alternative-medicine-and-health.com/therapy/mind-body.htm (accessed February 25, 2008).

6. H. Benson and T. Beary, "The Relaxation Response," *Psychiatry* 37 (1974): 37–46.

7. C. Dannecker and V. Wolf, "EMG-Biofeedback Assisted Pelvic Floor Muscle Training Is an Effective Therapy of Stress Urinary or Mixed Incontinence: A 7-Year Experience with 390 Patients," *Archives of Gynecology and Obstetrics* 273 (2005): 93–97.

8. Janet Kornblum, "Study: 25% of Americans Have No One to Confide In," *USA Today*, http://www.usatoday.com/news/nation/2006–6-22-friendship_x.htm (accessed retrieved February 25, 2008).

9. Sarah Ban Breathnach, *Simple Abundance: A Daybook of Comfort and Joy* (New York: Warner Books, 1995).

CHAPTER 8

1. Hsi Lai, *The Sexual Teachings of the Jade Dragon: Taoist Methods for Male Sexual Revitalization* (Rochester, Vt.: Destiny Books, 2002).

2. Gail Sheehy, *Sex and the Seasoned Woman: Pursuing the Passionate Life* (New York: Random House, 2006).

3. Sheehy, *Sex and the Seasoned Woman.*

4. Judith Wallerstsein and S. Blakeslee, *The Good Marriage: How and Why Love Lasts* (New York: Houghton Mifflin, 1995).

5. American Association of Retired Persons, "Sexuality at Midlife and Beyond: 2004 Update of Attitudes and Behaviors," *AARP The Magazine*, October 2005.

6. Ibid.

7. Ibid., 16.

8. Dona Caine, *When Benjamin Wants to Know: Family Conversations about the Facts of Life* (Chapel Hill, N.C.: Chapel Hill Press, 1995).

9. Rosemary Basson and J. Berman, "Report of the International Consensus Development Conference on Female Sexual Dysfunction: Definitions and Classifications," *Journal of Urology* 163 (2000): 888–93.

10. Lonnie Barbach, *Sex after 50: A Guide to Lifelong Sexual Pleasure* (video) (Ft. Lauderdale, Fla., 1991).

11. Ibid.

12. American Association of Retired Persons, "Sexuality and Beyond."

13. Ibid.

14. Paula Doress-Worters, *The New Ourselves Growing Older* (Gloucester: Peter Smith Publisher, 1996).

15. Barry Komisaruk and B. Whipple, *The Science of Orgasm* (Baltimore: Johns Hopkins University Press, 2006).

16. Rosemary Basson, "Women's Sexual Dysfunction: Revised and Expanded Definitions," *Canadian Medical Association Journal* 172, no. 10 (2005): 85–95.

17. North American Menopause Society, *3rd Edition Menopause Practice: A Clinician's Guide*, 3rd ed. (Cleveland: North American Menopause Society, 2007), 57.

18. Ibid., 61.

19. Basson, "Women's Sexual Dysfunction."

20. Edward Laumann and R. Michael, *Sex in America: A Definitive Study* (New York: Warner Books, 1994).

21. S. Plaut and A. Graziottrin, *Fast Facts—Sexual Dysfunction* (Oxford: Health Press, 2004).

22. Susan Rako, *The Hormone of Desire: The Truth about Testosterone, Sexuality, and Menopause* (New York: Three Rivers Press, 1996).

23. Robert Greene and Leah Feldon, *Perfect Balance* (New York: Three Rivers Press, 2005), 21.

24. Ibid., 166.

25. William Regelson, *The Super Hormone Promise* (New York: Pocket Books, 1997).

26. Marcelle Pick, "Adrenal Fatigue," http://www.womentowomen.com/adrenalfa tigue/dhea.aspx (accessed January 10, 2008).

27. Christiane Northrup, *The Wisdom of Menopause* (New York: Bantam Books, 2001), 119–23.

28. Zestra Laboratories, Charleston, S.C., http://www.zestra.com.

29. Greene and Feldon, *Perfect Balance.*

30. Eros Clitoral Stimulator, UroMetrics, Inc., Anoka, Minn., http://www.urometrics. com.

31. Greene and Feldon, *Perfect Balance.*

32. Komisaruk and Whipple, *The Science of Orgasm.*

33. R. C. Rosen, "Prevalence and Risk Factors of Sexual Dysfunction in Men and Women," *Current Psychiatry Reports,* no. 2 (2000), 189–95.

34. Komisaruk and Whipple, *The Science of Orgasm.*

35. Beverly Whipple and J. Perry, *The G Spot: And Other Discoveries about Human Sexuality* (New York: Random House, 1982).

36. Greene and Feldon, *Perfect Balance.*

37. Komisaruk and Whipple, *The Science of Orgasm.*

38. Ibid.

39. Basson, "Women's Sexual Dysfunction."

40. E. G. Friedrich, "Vulvarvestibulitis Syndrome," *Journal of Reproductive Medicine* 32, no. 2 (1987): 110–14.

41. K. J. Carlson and B. Miller, "The Maine Women's Health Study: Outcomes of Hysterectomy," *Obstetrics and Gynecology* 83 (1994): 556–85.

42. Laura Berman, *The Passion Prescription: Ten Weeks to Your Best Sex-Ever* (New York: Hyperion, 2005).

43. Ibid.

44. Ibid., 262–65.

45. Barbara Keesling, *The Good Girl's Guide to Bad Girls Sex* (New York: M. Evans and Company, 2001).

46. Northrup, *The Wisdom of Menopause.*

47. Harville Hendrix, *Getting the Love You Want: A Guide for Couples* (New York: Henry Holt, 1988).

48. Paul Shaffer, *Conflict Resolution for Couples: An Excellent Guide for Working through Relationship Issues* (Bloomington, Ind.: Author House, 2004).

49. Gary Chapman, *The Five Love Languages: How to Express Heartfelt Commitment to Your Mate* (Chicago: Northfield Publishing, 1995).

50. Laura Corn, *101 Nights of Great Romance* (Los Angeles: Park Avenue Publishers, 1996).

51. Edward Waring, *Enhancing Marital Intimacy: Through Facilitating Cognitive Self-Disclosure* (New York: Brunner/Mazel, 1988).

52. Janet Woititz, *Struggle for Intimacy* (Deerfield Beach, Fla.: Health Communications, 1985).

53. Jeremy Holmes, *John Bowlby and Attachment Theory: The Makers of Modern Psychotherapy* (New York: Brunner-Routledge, 1993).

54. William Masters and Virginia Johnson, *Human Sexual Response* (Boston: Little, Brown, 1966).

55. Helen Singer Kaplan, *The New Sex Therapy: Active Treatment of Sexual Dysfunctions* (New York: Brunner/Mazel, 1974).

56. Basson, "Women's Sexual Dysfunction."

57. Excerpts from "Genital Image Scale," in Berman, *The Passion Prescription;* Komisaruk and Whipple, *The Science of Orgasm.*

58. Excerpts from "Touch Yourself Exercise," in Keesling, *The Good Girl's Guide to Bad Girls Sex;* Sheehy, *Sex and the Seasoned Woman.*

59. Excerpts from "Genital Image Scale," Laura Berman, *The Passion Prescription: Ten Weeks to Your Best Sex—Ever* (New York: Hyperion, 2005). Reprinted with permission.

60. Keesling, *The Good Girl's Guide to Bad Girls Sex.*

61. Excerpts from "Touch Yourself Exercise," Barbara Keesling, *The Good Girl's Guide to Bad Girls Sex* (New York: M. Evans and Company, 2001). Reprinted with permission of the publisher M. Evans and Company.

62. Judy Kuriansky, *The Complete Idiot's Guide to Tantric Sex,* 2nd ed. (New York: Penguin, 2004).

63. American Association of Retired Persons, "Sexuality at Midlife and Beyond."

64. Corn, *101 Nights of Great Sex.*

65. Cory Silverberg, "Top Sexual Fantasies," May 29, 2007, http://sexuality.about.com/od/sexualityroleplay/a/top_sex_fantasy.html (accessed January 6, 2008).

66. Vanessa Burton, "Female Sex Fantasies," http://www.askmen.com/love/vanessa/27_love_secrets.html (accessed January 26, 2008).

67. Kathy Belge, "Top 10 Lesbian Sexual Fantasies," http://lesbianlife.about.com/od/lesbiansex/tp/Fantasies.htm (accessed January 26, 2008).

68. Emma Taylor and L. Sharkey, *Em & Lo's Sex Toy: An A-Z Guide to Bedside Accessories* (San Francisco: Chronicle Books, 2006).

69. American Association of Retired Persons, "Sexuality at Midlife and Beyond."

70. Michael Castleman, *Great Sex: A Man's Guide to the Secret Principles of Total-Body Sex* (New York: Rodale, 2004).

71. Taylor and Sharkey, *Em & Lo's Sex Toy.*

72. David Schnarch, *Constructing the Sexual Crucible: An Integration of Sexual and Marital Therapy* (New York: Norton, 1991).

73. Julia Heiman and J. LoPiccolo, *Becoming Orgasmic: A Sexual and Personal Growth Program for Women* (New York: Prentice Hall, 1988).

74. Sinclair Institute, "Better Sex Videos," http://www.bettersex.com.

75. Femme Productions, (800) 456-LOVE

76. William Cane, *The Art of Kissing* (New York: St. Martin's Griffin, 1995).

77. Corn, *101 Nights of Great Romance.*

INDEX

About the Author

DONA CAINE-FRANCIS, PMH-NP/CNS, is an ANCC Board Certified psychiatric mental health nurse practitioner, clinical nurse specialist, and AASECT certified sex therapist at Lake Norman outside of Charlotte, North Carolina. She is past president of the North Carolina Nurses Association and currently serves on the National Board for the American Nurses Association's Center for American Nurses. She is the author of *When Benjamin Wants to Know: Family Conversations about the Facts of Life* and *When Jessica Wants to Know* (forthcoming). She is a national speaker on "Speaking of Sex: How to Be an 'Askable Parent'" and "Sex and the Seasoned Woman: A Menopausal Survival Kit."